Finding Your Way Through Cancer

Finding
Your Way
Through
Cancer

An Expert Cancer Psychologist
Helps Patients and Survivors
Face the Challenges of Illness

*Based on the author's pioneering work
with more than 7,500 patients*

Andrew Kneier, PhD

CELESTIAL ARTS
Berkeley

To Caitlin and Michael

Published in the United States by Celestial Arts, an imprint of the
Crown Publishing Group, a division of Random House, Inc., New York.
www.crownpublishing.com
www.tenspeed.com

Celestial Arts and the Celestial Arts colophon are
registered trademarks of Random House, Inc.

Library of Congress Cataloging-in-Publication Data
Kneier, Andrew, 1945-
   Finding your way through cancer : an expert cancer psychologist helps
patients and survivors face the challenges of illness : based on the
author's pioneering work with more than 7,500 patients / Andrew Kneier.
      p. cm.
   Summary: "This guidebook delves into the top topics and concerns that
psychologist Andrew Kneier's 7,500 cancer patients have brought up
during therapy, from family to faith, suffering to resilience"—Provided
by publisher.
   Includes index.
   1. Cancer—Psychological aspects. 2. Cancer—Patients—Mental health.
3. Cancer—Treatment. 4. Psychotherapy. I. Title.
   RC271.P79K54 2010
   616.99'4—dc22
   2010015299

ISBN 978-1-58761-356-2

Printed in the United States of America

Design by Chloe Rawlins
Front cover photograph copyright © 2010
by Luca di Filippo/iStockPhoto

10 9 8 7 6 5 4 3 2 1

First Edition

Contents

Acknowledgments

I COULD LIST HERE THE NAMES of all the people with cancer who have confided in me over the course of my career. If you were to scan this list, your eyes might glaze over as one name blurred with the next. When I first met these people, they were just names to me as well. But soon I began to know and care about them as individuals, each with his or her own life history and each confronting the crosscurrents of suffering caused by cancer. They taught me about the challenges of living with cancer, and some taught me about dying of cancer and coming to terms with letting go. They honored me by not holding back, by telling me what it was really like for them to suffer in all the ways a person can suffer from a life-threatening illness. They also showed me what true resilience looks like, and how finding meaning can sustain a person through horrendous ordeals. They honored me by reaching out for my understanding and support and for whatever guidance I could offer. This book is my best but insufficient way of thanking them and honoring them in return.

A mental health professional who wants to work with cancer patients must be accepted and embraced by physicians who work in this field. I am indebted to the many physicians who did just that, starting with Drs. Lynn Spitler and Richard

Sagebiel, both of whom have devoted their careers to helping patients with malignant melanoma. They were the first to enlist my role in the care of their patients. Others followed at the University of California, San Francisco (UCSF), Comprehensive Cancer Center, especially Drs. Mohammed Kashani, Ernest Rosenbaum, Alan Glassberg, Laura Esserman, Peter Carrol, Thierry Jahan, Robert Allen, and Debu Tripathy. The cancer team at UCSF included other health care professionals who also supported my work there, especially Deborah Hamolsky, Barbara Buckley, Karen Stronach, and Rod Seeger. When I began at UCSF, I was welcomed and encouraged by the director of the Cancer Center, Dr. Frank McCormick.

After my time at UCSF, an extraordinary team of oncologists at the Sierra Nevada Memorial Hospital Comprehensive Community Cancer Center wholeheartedly included me in their whole-person approach to patient care. I am grateful to Drs. William Newsom, David Campbell, Richard Evans, David Kraus, and Brad Miller for welcoming me in this effort. The director of the Center, Ayse Turkseven, and the Center's oncology social worker, Rebecca Parsons, provided the leadership and support to make this possible. I am also indebted to Phil Genet for his generous grant to the Cancer Center to establish my role there.

To each person just listed, I extend my gratitude and appreciation. Had they not included me in the care of their patients, I would not have learned what I learned, and this book would not exist.

I am indebted to Lydia Temoshok, PhD, who chaired my dissertation and got me started in working with people suffering from metastatic melanoma.

My work at UCSF was generously supported by the Stephen Blumenthal Memorial Fund, and I am indebted to Sheryl Blumenthal and her family for making that happen. Generous funding was also provided by Phil Genet, Dr. Ernest Rosenbaum, Alan Baer, David Herschman, Brian Guance, and Deborah Huber. The UCSF Mount Zion Auxiliary and the UCSF Foundation played a key role in supporting my work.

I received invaluable feedback and encouragement from people with cancer who read earlier drafts of the essays in this collection. I especially thank Dorothea Nudelman, Frank Durham, Michelle Wilson, Karen Wagner, Linda Lachelt, Jana Peters, and Brady Williamson. Colleagues who read these drafts and contributed insight and encouragement included Dr. Jeff Kane, Mimi Roth, Peggy Blumberg, Dr. Neil Kostick, Melissa Horton, and Dr. John Curtis. Other indispensable readers included my wife, Katy, our daughter, Caitlin, my niece, Kristen Hill, and our valued friends David and Linda Palley. Kim Sagebiel, friend, novelist, and mentor to our children, guided and encouraged me through the publishing process.

When I was growing up, I aspired to emulate my older brother Gary. He is now in his late sixties and still going strong in his work as a clinical psychologist. He was so taken by my first drafts that he said he was proud to be my brother! This sweet remark became an impetus for me to continue working on these essays. He helped me improve them by offering pages of insightful comments born from his own clinical work and spiritual substance.

It was Dr. Elmer Grossman and his wife, Pam, who read the initial manuscript from cover to cover and took it upon themselves to encourage my eventual publisher, Celestial Arts, to take a serious look at my work. Had it not been for their intervention, this book would not exist—at least not in its present form, a form that was shaped and nurtured by those at Celestial Arts, most of all by my talented and wise editor, Lisa Westmoreland.

It took a village to make this book, and everyone mentioned here played a key role. If these essays prove helpful to those dealing with cancer, it is because I had a village teaching me and supporting me in my calling, If you are such a person, currently suffering from cancer, and find some guidance or comfort here, please give thanks in your heart, as I do, to all those who nurtured me along the way.

Introduction

A WOMAN WITH CANCER ONCE told me she found herself in a new world—a world where the sun, with its warmth and light, was eclipsed by something called cancer. The sky was gray like an overcast winter evening. She felt disoriented and lost. It was a world of cancer treatments, cancer anxiety, cancer dilemmas, and cancer challenges. Her former life was slipping away. She had embarked on a perilous new journey, she said, with no road map to guide her, no sure footing, and no confidence that she could make it through. Seeing her from the outside, you wouldn't know that she was in a new world. The sun was still in the sky, shining above her. But inside her mind and heart, a troubling preoccupation had set in. There was an in-your-face aspect to all the questions and anxieties that came with the news that she had cancer. Each morning her first thought was about cancer, about what to do and what would happen. Her dreadful thoughts would come and go like the tide of a dark ocean. This was her new journey, one defined with unrelenting uncertainty about her future existence.

The essays in this book are addressed to people in her situation. Like many people touched by cancer, perhaps you find yourself in a world like hers, launched against your will on a similar journey of unknown destination. Perhaps your suffering is similar as well: the suffering of anxiety, uncertainty, and the pressure to make the right moves on confusing terrain. You probably have taken the first steps and are now continuing to make your way as best you can as you confront one challenge after another. My aim in these essays is to help you along and help you through. We'll see if I can.

I will address you personally, assuming that either you are currently dealing with cancer or were treated for cancer some time ago and are now suffering from lingering side effects or the uncertainty of whether the cancer is gone for good. Whatever your situation may be, I believe you are suffering in your own personal ways and that the reality of your suffering is what led you to this book.

The suffering that cancer causes is our starting point. Underneath this suffering is your basic humanness. That is what makes you vulnerable to suffering in your body and mind, and what gives you a tenacity of spirit to bounce back and create meaning. Suffering has power, but you have power too. Your suffering happens to you, but, in some sense, *you* happen to *it*. You do not have to endure it passively or sheepishly.

Cancer causes people to suffer physically, emotionally, and spiritually. Your body can become a kind of battleground, with cancer on one side and medical treatments on the other. You are in the middle, and cancer and the fight against it can take a heavy toll. Often this physical suffering can overshadow everything else. But cancer also causes you to suffer emotionally. At its worst, it can feel like a tidal wave of fear and sorrow, of daunting challenges and impossible dilemmas, a tidal wave that drowns assumptions about the future—assumptions and plans that you used to make without a second thought. Cancer also throws a wrench in the works, in the precious patterns of your daily life and in the execution of plans and projects. We might call this the suffering of life disruption. And there can be spiritual suffering as well. You may try to make sense of your illness or search for a hidden reason or higher purpose behind it. The God of your faith and devotion may now seem silent, distant, and indifferent.

Much of the suffering that cancer causes is just plain pressure—the pressure or burden to get the right treatments, have the right attitude, and do the right things to maximize your chances. If your cancer progresses, you may blame yourself for not doing enough of the right things, and you may have the nagging, troubling feeling of letting others down. Your cherished relationships can suffer with strain and misunderstanding, and of course your loved ones have their own suffering to contend with (caused by *your* illness, creating guilt in you). You hate how your illness affects them, and you want to spare them. For their part, they want to be positive for your sake. Thus you may end up protecting each other from how you really feel. The closeness between you can suffer because of that. All of this and more is part of the package, part of the suffering caused by cancer.

For many people, there is a jolting demarcation—of their life before cancer (BC) and after diagnosis (AD). "It changes you forever." I have heard that countless times.

Too often the suffering cancer causes is minimized or trivialized as patients are told to keep a positive mental attitude. A positive attitude can help tremendously, but by itself it cannot cancel out your suffering. You need more than that to comfort and sustain you and to see you through. In these essays, I hope to offer more than just the encouragement to stay positive. I hope to help you find ways to honor and embrace your suffering as worthy of honest acknowledgment, attention, and respect.

As you probably know already, people who care about you tend to emphasize the positive or encouraging aspects of your diagnosis, treatment plan, test results, and so on. This is well intended, of course. But in the process, it can gloss over or downplay the worrisome or upsetting aspects, causing you to feel that you should not be too upset—perhaps not as upset as you really are. For example, if your scans are clear, someone may say that your cancer is behind you now, and that it's time to get your life back. You may know that the other shoe could drop at any moment, and if that happened, you'd be staring death in the face. This is the reality that you are living with, day in and day out, and it may seem that others don't get it.

I think we should call a spade a spade when it comes to the inherent suffering that cancer causes. It is good, I believe, to face up to things the way they are. It is good for others to see, and for you to know, that you have valid reasons for how you feel.

When I discuss your emotional distress in the pages to follow, I want to do so in a way that validates it and helps you to understand it more fully and deeply, in all its dimensions and nuances. You may wonder what benefit can come from that. When you were a child and skinned your knee, for example, did it help if there was a caring adult around who knew that it hurt, who let you cry as much as you needed, and who just held you until you were ready to be on your way? And what kind of help was that, if not the help of feeling that your injury was real, your tears were valid, and comfort was at hand for as long as you needed? You were helped to feel these things about your injury because someone else was there to validate the reality of your experience. Perhaps this person also knew the context of this injury, how it came on top of some other recent hurt. When that was acknowledged, you may have cried even more, but felt even more understood and better after this harder cry.

Although we start with suffering, we need not end there. I mentioned earlier your tenacity of spirit. You have immense resources inside yourself, and hopefully all around you, to respond with compassion toward yourself and with power toward your suffering. Perhaps you have heard of Viktor Frankl's book *Man's Search for Meaning*. Many of his fellow inmates in a Nazi concentration camp were able to turn their suffering into a personal triumph through a strength of will to endure unimaginable brutality and to refuse to give in or give up. Think for a minute about whether this idea might help you— the idea that you can turn your suffering into a personal triumph by virtue of how you relate to it and what you do with it.

Your suffering is physical, and in that sense it is what it is. But the emotional impact is not a given, independent of your thoughts and attitudes about it. I am thinking of a woman who suffered horribly by losing a breast, being burned, being poisoned, and losing her hair. But she felt proud (rather than ashamed) of her bald head and scarred body because it showed the price she was willing to pay in order to live. Her suffering did not define her as a pitiful creature. It did not have that power over her. She was the one who dictated the meaning of her suffering, not the other way around. The same is true for you.

You are in charge of what things mean.

Cancer can do hideous things to your body, but you can be in charge of what it does to your soul or inner self. You can be scared but not intimidated, singled out, or victimized. It is time for your best self to come forth and to sustain you through all the physical horrors that cancer can dish out.

It may be presumptuous to say I want to help. After all, you are the one dealing with cancer. I am just a psychologist— but one who has years of experience listening to thousands of people with cancer describe their suffering and the dimensions of it that are private, subtle, and often insidious. I have been moved, inspired, and educated. I have learned about common dilemmas, common fears, and common psychological struggles. I have discovered ways of thinking about and working through these issues. I am grateful for all I have learned. If there is wisdom in these pages, it comes from ordinary people like yourself who have made this journey before you. My goal now is to share this wisdom, passed from them to you.

People with cancer have also shown me the phenomenal internal resources that reside in our nature for coping, resilience, and finding meaning. I read about this in college, but until I had the privilege of working with people who had cancer, listening to them, and observing their personal power in the face of suffering, I had no clue really, no real understanding or appreciation of what we are made of. The fairy tale about turning straw into gold speaks to a capacity in the human spirit that I have witnessed firsthand.

I have also learned firsthand about the unshakable fear that can grip you when you first hear you might have cancer. This happened to me in my late twenties. Fortunately, I had a therapist to help me through this horrible time as I went from one test to another. It turned out to be a false alarm. I then became a therapist myself with the hope of helping others as I had been helped.

In these essays I will also draw on what I have learned in my studies in psychology, philosophy, and religion. Before I became a psychologist, I was on the road to becoming a professor of religion, and I was especially interested in the philosophy of religion. Although that doesn't make me an expert, my experiences as a therapist have taught me how these disciplines can be relevant to people who are dealing with cancer. From philosophy, I know the importance of perspective, of taking stock of the bigger picture, as we also take stock of our own plight and the nuances of meaning it contains. From theology, I have learned about the importance of one's religious beliefs or spirituality in dealing with human suffering and adversity.

Each essay in this collection stands on its own. You can read them in any order you wish. You might just read those of particular interest to you. That would be fine. My aim is to help, not to burden you with more reading than you feel ready to tackle at this time.

To help you decide which essays are most relevant to your personal situation, I offer the following synopses of what the essays are about.

Cancer and Your Life Story

In our minds, we all construct the "story of our lives" based on our life experiences, both good and bad. When we think about the meaning of our lives, we are thinking about the meaning of this story. When cancer enters, this story is changed. A new chapter begins, and its meaning will stem partly from your life story up to that point and partly from how you respond to your illness. Whatever meaning your illness carries, it will have an effect on your emotions and behavior. Your perception of a negative meaning behind your cancer (such as punishment for things you felt guilty about) can make you pessimistic and depressed. I give two case examples to illustrate this point. In each case, once the person saw how his or her life story was creating a negative meaning, they were able to respond in more positive ways and thus create a more positive meaning. How do you see your illness? Is it consistent with a negative theme in your life story or does it offer an opportunity to change your story in positive ways? That's what this essay is about.

Family Matters

Cancer is a family illness in the sense that it disrupts family life and causes emotional upset in each family member. Many families seem to conspire, in a way, to keep the lid on, protect each other emotionally, and carry on as before. Although well intended, this approach can get in the way of a deeper emotional closeness within a family. This essay takes up the fear, sorrow, and guilt that can occur for all family members, and how these emotions are often handled in families. I also discuss the difficult issue of what children should be told (or not told) about a grown-up's illness and some principles that apply to the content and timing of these disclosures.

Learning from Your Emotions

Cancer has an emotional impact on everyone. Although it may seem that one person's emotions are pretty much the same as another's, emotional responses are actually unique to each individual. They are based on very personal thoughts and carry personal meanings that stem from each person's past experience. There is much to be learned from your emotions—about yourself, what is important to you, your personal emotional history, and your appraisal of your situation and the significant people involved. In this essay I give three case examples to illustrate these points. This essay is about self-exploration and self-discovery, using your emotions as a starting point.

Mastering Anxiety

Everyone who has cancer has anxiety too, to varying degrees at various times. If you think about how you are dealing with anxiety, you'll probably recognize certain approaches or strategies that have worked for you in the past and that are consistent with your personality. I know many people with cancer who have made a concerted effort to master their anxiety. They have developed many effective approaches and techniques, and I share those in this essay in hopes that these approaches can also help you.

Giving Attitude to Cancer

Right now, as you read this, you have a certain attitude or approach to your illness. It is probably not an attitude you deliberately chose after weighing the pros and cons of other options. It might be more accurate to say that you *find yourself* with an attitude or approach that seems right for you. But where did this attitude come from? What gave rise to it in this situation? What does it say about you, your strengths and weaknesses, your personal history, and how you relate to suffering? In this essay, I hope to help you reflect on these questions with an aim toward embracing all the ways your attitude serves you well while also considering possible pitfalls and whether another approach could actually be better for you. I do this by discussing five attitudes that commonly arise in people who have cancer.

Five Existential Dilemmas

This essay discusses five dilemmas that most people with cancer confront, in various ways and at various times. How do you balance, for example, being optimistic but also realistic? How do you give your illness the attention it deserves while not letting it take over your life? How do you allow yourself to be justifiably upset over your illness while also keeping in mind that many others are worse off? And finally, how do you allow yourself to feel rotten when you are hurting while not giving in to sickness too readily? Most people with cancer want to have the "right" emotional reaction, but it is not readily apparent what that reaction should be. I hope this essay will help you resolve these dilemmas in a way that is right for you.

God and Suffering

This essay is relevant to those of you who are searching for comfort and guidance from your religious faith or spirituality. This search invariably runs up against some troubling questions. Why, for example, does God allow innocent people to suffer? How does your illness fit into God's plan or purpose? Why does God seem so distant, silent, and even indifferent as you suffer from cancer? If God can't or won't intervene, then what does it make sense to pray for? In the philosophy of religion, the deistic tradition provides a view of God's relation to the world that can help with these questions. It points to the spirit of God in each person, a spirit that can be called upon to help when dealing with cancer. In this context, I discuss five things worth praying for.

On Coming to Terms with the Possibility of Death

One way to have a peaceful death is to come to terms with it before your illness advances to a terminal stage. Many people with cancer do that, especially if their prognosis is poor. In this essay I discuss how patients I know have come to feel a sense of acceptance about their eventual death. Most of this discussion is based on interviews I conducted, as part of a study, with patients who were relatively young and had a poor prognosis. Many thoughts and emotions helped them in this process. If you are struggling with this issue—wanting somehow to feel reconciled to dying, when the time comes, but not knowing how to get there—it may help to learn how other people with cancer have done that.

Cancer as a Gift?

Cancer, of course, is not a gift. But for many people, having cancer has actually enriched their lives in certain respects, and these patients often refer to it as a gift. In this essay I discuss five ways that cancer can be (in part) a positive experience, and I give many examples from people I know. Cancer can be a wake-up call to pay attention to what really matters and to live with greater appreciation and gratitude. It can help you to live more fully in the present moment. It can make you more aware of how much you are loved and valued. Often, in response to cancer, a person's best self comes to the fore. Cancer can also lead to a deepening of a person's faith or spirituality. If you have not yet encountered these positive aspects, perhaps my discussion and examples will help bring them to life in your own experience.

My Interrupted Life: Jenny's Story

Each person's experience with cancer is completely unique, and there is no one right way to go through it. This is one unique story: the story of Jenny, a remarkable forty-two-year-old woman with colon cancer. Her story is told in the first person, constructed from transcripts of our therapy sessions, her journal entries, and my notes from our sessions and the support group meetings she attended. If you read her story, you will see that she is remarkable in her ability to face hard realities head-on. I think you will be impressed by her ability to articulate the conflicts and dilemmas that bounced around in her mind and may be bouncing around in yours. Her story brings to life many of the themes addressed in these essays, and it also reflects the individual and personal nature of each person's experience. (My wife said everyone should read this story first!)

I use patients' names in the essays in this collection, but these names are fictitious and I have changed other identifying information to protect the privacy of those who have shared their experience with me. In all cases, this sharing has been deeply personal, and I have been honored to be on the receiving end of it. I have tried to honor these patients in turn by sharing with you what I have learned from them.

ONE

Cancer and Your Life Story

MARY HAD BEEN ABUSED all her life, first physically as a child, then sexually in her teenage years, and later in an abusive marriage. She said that being abused was more or less the story of her life. When she was diagnosed with breast cancer, it felt like one more instance of abuse, echoing the sexual and marital abuse in her past. In her mind, it confirmed something awful about herself and her life—namely, that she was fated to be abused. "It's not at all surprising that I should get breast cancer," she said. "It totally fits." Seeing her cancer in that way made it all the more depressing.

Stephanie had a similar life history, but the story in her mind was much different. "It seems like I've always been a target for people's anger," she said, "so I've always needed to be strong and fight back." When she was diagnosed with ovarian cancer, she felt that once again she needed to resist. She did so with enormous tenacity, pursuing the most aggressive treatments and making positive changes in her health habits.

These stories illustrate two concepts: first, that we all construct "the story of our lives" based on our life experience, both good and bad; second, that new problems we encounter—from serious illness to divorce—carry certain meanings depending on how they fit into our life story. The life-narrative approach to psychotherapy is based on this idea—that our life story is the basis for attributing meaning to life events and for creating new meanings when necessary.

Putting a new problem in the context of our life story allows us to better understand the emotions or conflicts that arise. If this new problem is cancer, it could feel consistent with a certain theme in one's story, as it did for Mary and Stephanie. More important, the story affects how each person acts in response to the illness. Mary responded as a victim because that's the character she had created for herself in her life story. Stephanie responded like a warrior because her self-created character is that of a combatant who can rise to any challenge.

Think about your own life story for a minute, from birth to the time you were diagnosed. What are the main chapters and turning points? Who are the main characters? Is there a main plot or theme? In other words, what is the story about? What does it say about your life—and about *you*? How has it shaped your identity—the way you see or define yourself?

Now cancer enters your story. You can feel blindsided by it. Certainly it disrupts the story, perhaps turning things upside down. But how does it fit in? What does it say about you, or about your life's journey, that now you have cancer to contend with? Many people with cancer have told me, "I'm trying to figure out what it all means." When you try to figure out what it means to you, you're thinking about cancer in the *context* of your life story, even if you aren't aware of it at first. You may feel that your cancer doesn't carry any meanings, hidden or otherwise. You may be right about that, but certainly your *response* to your illness says something about your identity and life story. Each person reacts to a cancer diagnosis in his or her own personal way. Your reaction carries personal meanings. It could be consistent, for example, with how you have reacted to adversity in the past. But it could also show that a different (and perhaps more positive) aspect of your personality is coming to the fore. Your reaction could be a way of breaking new ground in your life story and in how you define yourself.

For example, Steve, a man with lung cancer, felt that he was always on his own when dealing with life's challenges. "No one has really helped me along," he said. This was a dominant theme in his life story. His cancer diagnosis, however, became a turning point for him. Instead of thinking it was up to him to figure out what to do about it, he decided to place himself in the hands of his doctors. "It's time to trust that others can help me," he said. This capacity and willingness to trust did not come easily for him, but he felt it was long overdue.

As we construct a life story, the key events in our lives are the raw material we draw upon. These events, however, do not by themselves tell a story. We are the authors of our story, and we determine what things mean. We are meaning-creating creatures. Even if, consciously, we can't quite nail down what something means, we always see things in terms of a narrative we've constructed for ourselves. Cognitive psychology studies the role of our left-brain activity in creating subjective meanings and then reacting to events based on these meanings, even though we may not be consciously aware of them. When people with cancer become depressed, it is often because of underlying depressing *thoughts* about the meaning of their illness.

Over the years, many people have talked with me about the meaning of their cancer or how they were responding to it. Here are some common themes.

Cancer as a Message

People often see a message in their cancer. It speaks to them about a change that is necessary in their lifestyle, relationships, or basic life approach. I knew a man with colon cancer who always felt driven to accomplish more, thinking that what he had was not enough. He saw his cancer as a message to slow down and count his blessings. A woman with breast cancer felt competitive with other women, tending to regard them as rivals. When she was diagnosed, however, she began thinking of other women with breast cancer as allies or "sisters," and this helped her let her guard down with other women, including her female oncologist. She saw her cancer as a message to be more trusting of women. Often people feel that it took something like cancer to make a point, to force them to learn a positive lesson. "I needed to learn to be more grateful for what I have," a patient told me, "and cancer is certainly teaching me that."

An Opportunity for Change

For many people, cancer is not just a message or lesson. It's actually an *opportunity* for positive change. Seizing this opportunity becomes part of their response to their illness. Someone who had been very self-sufficient, for example, can respond by reaching out for support. Someone who had been very private about his emotions can respond by being more open. Someone who had tended to defer to authority figures can respond by asking questions and seeking second opinions.

Cancer Balances Things Out

Sometimes people feel, before getting cancer, that they've had a kind of charmed life. They feel exceptionally fortunate, especially in light of all the hardship and suffering in the world around them. They have a nagging worry in the back of their minds that something bad is bound to happen to balance things out. "I've had more than my fair share of good luck," one person told me.

Cancer as Punishment

Our culture is influenced by the Judeo-Christian tradition, a tradition that often sees illness as punishment for sin. In the Book of Job, for example, the countless sufferings that befell him implied that he was a sinner. He protested that he was a very righteous person and therefore did not *deserve* all these calamities. No one has led a perfect life or always lived up to his or her ideals. Some people feel guilty for neglecting their duties or responsibilities. Others feel that something good came their way at the expense of someone else. These are some of the reasons people feel guilty and thus wonder whether their cancer is punishment or a price they must now pay for something in their past.

A Fighting Spirit

Some people feel powerless to influence the course of their illness. It is more common, however, for people to see it as a challenge that requires a strong fighting spirit. Perhaps they have been timid when confronted with hardships in the past, but this time, in response to cancer, they stand up and fight back with a newfound tenacity of spirit, refusing to be intimidated by it.

Take a moment and consider whether any of these themes fit into your life story—or how you may want them to. If you can see your cancer as an opportunity for change, making this change could be a way of promoting your health—whether mental or physical—in response to cancer. Or if you've been subconsciously viewing cancer as a punishment or a way to balance things out, it might be helpful to realize that cancer does not really carry any such meanings.

Themes embedded in your life story can also be embedded in your response to cancer. Kevin, whose story follows, came to see how his reaction to his illness was influenced by such themes—themes that were not really rational. Once he saw that, he was able to make some positive changes in his life and in his story.

Kevin and Malignant Melanoma

Kevin was the only child in an unhappy marriage. His parents divorced when he was five. After that he rarely saw his father. He said his mother was very depressed after the divorce. He had vivid memories of her crying on the living room sofa. He would sit next to her, not knowing how to console her.

When he was seven his mother took him to his father's apartment to ask him to return home. "Just tell him I want him back," she said. She implied that this would carry more weight coming from Kevin. He was to be her emissary. She drove him to the apartment where his father was living with another woman, told him the apartment number, and sent him on his impossible mission. He rang the doorbell but no one answered. He had mixed feelings as he walked back to the car. He felt relieved for being let off the hook, but he also felt guilty that he had to deliver bad news to his mother. "I hated having to tell her that no one was home," he recalled.

His mother worked part-time and was home in the afternoons. He remembered other kids staying after school to play soccer, but he always felt that he needed to rush home. His mother would be there waiting. He said it always cheered her up when he'd walk through the door. "I'm home, Mom!" he would yell.

Kevin got good grades in high school. He dated only a few times. He was interested in sports, but did not try out for any teams, continuing to come home right after school. After he graduated he attended a local junior college and continued to live at home. He wanted to transfer to a state university after that, but it was about eight hours away. He was interested in chemistry and wanted to do research in the pharmaceutical industry. Instead, he stayed home and got a job at a local pharmacy. When he was twenty-three, his mother remarried and moved into a new house. Kevin continued his college education and earned a bachelor's degree in chemistry, but he decided to become a clinical nurse specialist instead of doing pharmaceutical research. He was twenty-nine years old when I met him. He had been married for about two years.

I met Kevin about a month after he was diagnosed with malignant melanoma. It had originated on his back and had spread to his lymph nodes, which were surgically removed. There was no evidence of any other metastases. He was told there was a significant risk of recurrence, but that no additional treatments were warranted. He just had to wait, watch for a recurrence, and get periodic checkups.

What struck me about Kevin was that he showed no emotional upset or worry over his diagnosis. He told his mother that he was fine. He did not want her to worry. He was referred to me because his doctor thought he was depressed. He admitted he sometimes felt blue, but was not sure why. It was not his melanoma, he said. Work was fine. "I don't know," he shrugged. Then he said, "Well, my wife bugs me at times." I asked him to explain why, but he resisted and said something like "No one is perfect" and "All told, it's really okay." He said his wife was eager to have a baby but he wasn't sure whether he wanted children. He said his wife was upset about that.

What can we make of all this so far? Kevin had essentially told me certain chapters of his life story up to that point, although neither of us had referred to it as a story. I asked him to think about his life as a story, a story that started long ago and continued to the present. "What would that story be about?" I asked. He took a few moments to think about that. He then said, "Well, it's about my mother, and always having to worry about her." He might have identified many other story lines in his history, but this was the one that came to mind. He added that he felt responsible for making her happy. We can see why he would say that. He tried to console her on the sofa when she was crying. He'd rush home after school to cheer her up. Toward the end of this discussion he mentioned his wife. "I don't like it when she gets depressed," he said. "It's like my mother all over again."

His unemotional response to his illness seems consistent with a theme in his life story—namely, the obligation to attend to the emotions of *others* instead of paying attention to his own needs. This orientation toward others was established in his mind at an early age with his mother, which laid down a template for subsequent relationships. In her depression, his mother was not able to focus on young Kevin's emotional needs—his need for comfort and support, for example, in losing contact with his father, or his need to have a life of his own by staying after school to play with his friends. Although she probably did not do this intentionally, the message conveyed by her behavior was that her emotional needs mattered more than his.

Because he was living in limbo now, not knowing whether he was cured or whether his melanoma would return and prove fatal, we can imagine many normal feelings of fear and upset. But he was not supposed to attend to those emotions. Instead, he put on a happy face to protect his mother from worry.

Kevin felt responsible for making his mother happy partly because he inferred that he had the ability to do that. His mother was convinced that if he appeared as her emissary, his plea to his dad would carry weight. This implied that he was a powerful young boy. These experiences cemented in his mind an awful belief that became a burden for many years hence—

the belief that he had the power and the responsibility to rescue his mother. He was only seven.

I also learned that Kevin had been thinking of divorcing his wife before he was diagnosed. He described her as overly needy and dependent on him. He said she had almost no friends of her own or any outside activities or interests. "It seems like I am the center of her world," he said, "and it's a big burden." He admitted that he was not really ambivalent about having children; he was ambivalent about his marriage and having children *with her*. Not surprisingly, he felt guilty about wanting to leave his wife. He imagined that she would be totally devastated. He also felt that it was his duty to take care of needy women (we know how that originated) and therefore felt that leaving his wife would be shirking his duty.

From his past, he felt guilty for failing to make his mother happy, and in his current situation, he felt guilty for wanting to be free from his wife. Thus, when he was diagnosed, he interpreted it as punishment *and* as a warning to "cease and desist" his forbidden desire to leave his wife. After his diagnosis he no longer wanted a divorce, he told me. Instead, he said that he was trying to focus on his wife's positive characteristics and on the good aspects of their relationship. He imagined that his change of heart would prevent his melanoma from recurring. You can see the logic of this strategy. If his melanoma was punishment for wanting to leave his wife, he would no longer need to be punished if he stopped doing the thing he was being punished for.

We now have a better understanding of why Kevin did not seem worried about his illness and why he was depressed. It was depressing to believe that he was guilty of a crime (when the crime in question was a legitimate desire to be free of a burdensome obligation to make needy and dependent women happy), that he was being punished for this crime by contracting a life-threatening illness, and that the only way to be safe from a recurrence was to negate his legitimate desires. After his diagnosis, Kevin also started to be more attentive to his mother. He called her more often and even invited her and her husband to join him and his wife on a vacation. His effort to be more involved in his mother's life, and thus to make her happy, was part of his strategy—explained by his life story—to keep melanoma away.

I worked with Kevin for about two years. During this time he constructed a new way of thinking about his life and the meaning of his illness. In the new story, he saw his life as a struggle—a struggle to pry himself loose from the burdensome and unfair duty that had been imposed by the circumstances of his childhood, and a struggle to keep alive the hope and striving for a happier life, a life that was a gift for him to enjoy (as opposed to a life devoted only to the happiness of others). The struggle that characterized his life was also about knowing, validating, and expressing his own emotions and needs. In this story, his melanoma took on new meanings. It created powerful emotions that could not be denied. He needed something like this to happen, he said—something so frightening and so traumatic that it would push through the prohibition on his emotional life. He needed something that, in other words, would force him to reevaluate his life story and pay attention to his own emotions.

The other new meaning for him was a warning that he needed to get on with his own life. The message in his melanoma was stark and powerful: if he continued to deny and repress his emotional needs, and if he continued to live with the internal stress of duty, burden, and guilt, he would be jeopardizing his very existence. Often people are cured of melanoma because of a vigorous immune response, and the immune system can be weakened by the repression of emotion and by feeling trapped in a stressful situation. He therefore felt that staying in an unhappy and burdensome marriage was *not* the safe thing to do; it was actually dangerous. In his therapy, Kevin worked on all these issues related to guilt and emotional repression. He became more aware of his real feelings about many troubling events in his life story, including his melanoma. He came to feel that he had a right to be happy, and he eventually left his unhappy marriage and began building a new life story for himself.

Laura and Breast Cancer

Laura was the youngest of three children. She told me her childhood was happy and uneventful. Her family life was very peaceful, she said. She explained that everyone seemed to get along. She could not recall any serious arguments or emotional outbursts. She thought her parents were compatible, although they seldom expressed physical affection in front of their children.

Laura recalled a Halloween party she was invited to when she was about ten years old. It registered in her memory because it was very upsetting. She could not decide whether she wanted to go as a clown, a princess, a ghost, or something else entirely. Her mother took her to a costume store. There were lots of good costumes to choose from, but Laura was at a loss. She was so indecisive that she did not attend the party. It was not so much that she *decided* not to go; rather, it was more or less by default that she would not attend the party because she could not decide on a costume.

Laura did well in school without really having to try very hard. Her high school offered many extracurricular activities, but she could not decide on any of them. It reminded her of the Halloween experience. Once again she felt paralyzed. A friend persuaded her to join the debate team. She recalled that the topics to be debated were assigned to them, along with the side of the issue (pro or con) they had to argue. She remembered this detail because it was so greatly relieving to her.

After high school she could not decide whether to attend college. She considered working, but had no strong preference for any one job. Would she stay at home or get a place of her own? These decisions were overwhelming to her. She felt paralyzed, just as before. "I had no inner feeling about what I wanted to do or be," she told me.

She had a steady boyfriend during her senior year, and they got married after graduation. Her marriage more or less solved the problem of what she would do after high school. Her husband worked in a family business that was very successful. Money was not a problem, and Laura did not need to work. She spent the first year of their marriage fixing up their home and then became pregnant. She said she did not really decide to have a child; her pregnancy was an accident. She enjoyed being a mother, however. "It gave a focus to my life," she told me. A few years later she and her husband decided to have another child. She said it was the obvious thing to do so their first child would have a sibling to play with. She remained happily married during the following years and enjoyed raising her children and being a wife and mother.

Laura was diagnosed with breast cancer when she was only thirty-four years old. It was an aggressive tumor that had invaded the lymph nodes under her arm. Her scans showed no evidence of metastases, but chemotherapy was warranted nonetheless. She was told that her five-year survival chances were about 60 percent.

I met Laura about one month after she was diagnosed. What she told me about the meaning of her diagnosis was remarkable. She felt that it was a dramatic message to get in touch with her inner self and to decide for the first time what she really wanted to do with her life. She had figured this out on her own. From my therapy notes, she said something like this: "All my life I have felt empty inside, like I had no inner guide to help me decide things. I've just gone along with the flow, like a cork in a river. When there was a fork in the river, the current took me this way or that. I wish I had been a boat with a rudder, the captain of my ship. Then I could have decided things." She was talking, of course, about a dominant theme in her life story. This story line was about to change.

Her diagnosis had concentrated her mind like nothing else ever had. She was very clear about some essential points. It was imperative that she discover her inner self, the person she really was, and to be true to herself. "I am here for a reason," she said, "and I need to know what that is."

I asked if she felt she had *needed* a wake-up call of this magnitude. She agreed, but not in the sense that some agent or force had sent her what she needed. Nor did she think she developed cancer because she needed to get in touch with her true self. She was very down-to-earth and did not attribute complicated causal factors to her diagnosis. The message in her cancer was not *from* anybody or anything. It was just there, shouting out to her. When I asked why a cancer diagnosis would have this effect on her, her answer was very straightforward. She said the cancer could kill her, and it brought home the fact that she had one and only one life to live and that she did not want to waste it being a cork in a river. It was as simple as that.

But it was also as profound as that. It's a simple and yet deep truth that we should not waste our lives. The notion that we have a life, and that it's for something or about something, is enormously compelling. We cannot prove this to be true, but we *feel* it to be true.

In my work with Laura we explored the origins of her inde-
cisiveness. She thought it had something to do with family
dinners when she was young. She said they were peaceful and
polite, but also somewhat boring and stifling. "It seemed like
nobody had any feelings about anything," she said. On the
surface, her family life seemed content, but it troubled Laura
that they were not really emotionally close. I wondered if she
conformed to the family norm of not expressing emotion as a
way of being close to her family. This touched a chord. In her
mind, one way of having some semblance of closeness was to
be like everyone else, to be emotionally empty in a way. If she
expressed her feelings, she feared it would only alienate her
from the others. So she learned not to have any strong emotions. She regarded them as dangerous and threatening to her
bond with her family. At one point she said, "I didn't want to
rock the boat, so I must have turned off my emotions." I had no
way of knowing if this was really necessary. Perhaps others in
the family would have welcomed some emotional heat. Nonetheless, this was how she sized things up—that being emotionally flat was the norm, and she was supposed to be that way
too—and thus began a theme in her life story.

Over the course of her therapy, Laura realized that she
wanted to be an interior decorator and eventually own an
interior decorating business. She found that she enjoyed decorating her own home and that she had a special talent for it.
The suburb where they lived was growing, and she thought
there would be an increasing need for decorating help. She
also thought she could pursue this career and stay actively
involved in raising her children. She knew she'd need to go
to school first, but was undaunted by that. Informed by the
meaning of her life story, she began writing a new chapter—on
purpose this time.

There is an old saying that we should not die with our music
inside. This saying spoke volumes to Laura because her aspi-

rations and talents (her music) had been locked inside until her cancer diagnosis prompted—or rather, compelled—them to the surface.

Laura's story illustrates how positive meaning can be found in one's illness. I ran into her at a cancer center event about a year after we had stopped our weekly therapy sessions. Her cancer had not recurred. She wanted to tell me that, but she wanted to make another point. She said her cancer experience had been an awful ordeal but that something positive had come out of it for her. "It made me find myself," she said. Cancer had forced her to analyze her life story, change the character and role assigned to her, and rewrite the plot in keeping with her true self.

When Kevin and Laura stepped back from key events in their lives and saw a story there, certain themes emerged that gave meaning to their illness. What they needed to do, what they needed in their lives, became clear to them. If necessary, this can be true for you, too. Think about your life as a story and see what themes jump out. Do these themes give a certain meaning to your illness? Just ask yourself: What does it mean that I developed cancer? What does it mean that I have reacted in the ways I have? You might jot down your answers to ponder them. Do these meanings guide and empower you in ways that affirm a positive inner truth about your life and about yourself? If not, can you find alternative meanings that do that?

You did not ask for this new chapter in your life, the one about cancer and you. But it's here now, and it needs to be written by you. Don't let past themes in your life story dictate meanings that only make you feel worse—perhaps more alone, more trapped, or more helpless than you really are. Try to compose positive meanings that capture a hidden truth about yourself, that capture the music inside, as Kevin and Laura were able to do.

TWO

Family Matters

IN MANY RESPECTS, cancer happens to your entire family. The impact on them loops back to have an impact on you. You might try to control this impact by downplaying your suffering. That could be a mistake, as I will discuss. It can go the other way too. Members of your family may try to control the impact of their emotions on you by hiding those emotions. Or they may minimize the seriousness of your illness, or only emphasize the reasons to be hopeful and optimistic. These ploys, while common and understandable in their intent, can also be a mistake. You want your family's support, but what does support really mean? Does it mean being positive, or does it mean being emotionally close? There can be a big difference. If you feel guilty, it may seem to make no sense; and your loved ones can feel guilty too, especially about their resentment. And what about your children? What should you tell them? To protect them, you may downplay the seriousness of your cancer, or not even call it cancer. Although this approach is based on your love for them, it could be a mistake to protect them too much. We have lots to consider here. Let's get started.

Family Fears

A cancer diagnosis scares people—namely, you and everyone who loves you. That goes without saying. But you don't want your loved ones to be afraid, and they don't want you to be afraid. To this end, discussions about your illness in the family are likely to focus mostly on the positive aspects. This is very common, but there can be some downsides. For one, your effort to be positive could require you to suppress your true emotions. Thus you would not have the *outlet* you need for your own fears. This kind of suppression can cause depression and compromise the immune system.

Another downside concerns the nature of support. Your family may try to support you by offering encouragement. A family member might say, for example, that you'll be fine, they just know it. But if this glosses over the true seriousness of your illness—namely, the real possibility that you *won't* be fine—it could feel unsupportive. Your family may convey that they are with you in your fight against cancer. On the face of it, that sounds supportive. But this support would be more meaningful, I think, if they also acknowledged (instead of skirting the issue) what all of you are fighting *against*—specifically, the threat posed to your life.

More than anything else, I believe, support involves emotional closeness and therefore a sharing of all the emotions that come with cancer. It means you and your family are scared together, have hope together, and are linked arm-in-arm in a positive plan for the future. You share your true fears, and your loved ones see the validity of those fears while also sharing their own. In other words, *your shared emotions are the ground of your closeness.* Let's think about how to achieve that.

At first, you may hold back from expressing your emotions if you think it will make others feel worse. It seldom does, however. I have met with thousands of couples wherein one member had cancer. It was very common, for example, for husbands to protect their wives by downplaying their fears. When they admitted to this, their wives were quick to reassure them, saying something like this: "Honey, I'm scared too. Hearing that you are scared doesn't make me feel worse. It makes me feel closer to you."

I doubt your loved ones want to be protected and kept at arm's length. When you act positive and upbeat when you really don't feel that way, you are essentially keeping them out of your inner sanctum where your true emotions reside.

If you sense that those unspoken fears have become an "elephant in the room" that everyone sees but no one acknowledges, you can begin to open things up by saying to your family something like this: "You know, cancer is scary for all of us, and that's OK. We can face that together and say how we really feel." You'll find your own words, but I think you get the idea.

Sometimes we worry so much about the needs and feelings of others that we lose sight of our own. Suppose you are feeling upset and needing support, but you *assume* your family needs you to be positive and does not want to be burdened by your emotional needs. In this situation, you may be inclined to keep quiet about your feelings and needs because, in your mind, protecting your family's emotions comes first.

In some situations, of course, it is good to put your own needs aside and instead focus on someone else. Many of us, however, do this automatically by force of habit, by the force of a compelling belief derived from countless experiences in our childhood—experiences that presented a skewed message about whose rights and needs mattered most. If this applies to you, and if you've come to believe that you should always give priority to others, then you've been going through life with your antennae tuned to the emotional world around you—a world populated by other people with overriding emotional needs. In the process, of course, your own legitimate needs and emotions may not have gotten the attention they deserve.

Sometimes people have strong emotional needs that are sealed off from their conscious awareness; thus, they don't *know* what they really need. Think about your own experience when you were young. Did it pay to know and disclose your needs because of the support you received? Did you have a parent who had emotional reserves just for you, as opposed to being depleted by the demands of raising a family? Perhaps at times it backfired to disclose your needs because it seemed to bother or inconvenience others, leaving you feeling alone, scolded, and guilty for your feelings. If this was your reality when you were young, then the safest strategy was to protect yourself from being hurt by warding off these needs, keeping them unknown to yourself and others. I hope that your reality now is more supportive.

Family Sorrow

Fear is one thing; sorrow is another. It's more complicated because it can smack of self-pity or feeling sorry for yourself, which have negative connotations. Paradoxically, it's natural to feel sorry for someone else who has cancer, but to feel the same toward yourself can seem self-absorbed and lacking in perspective (because so many others are worse off). What about feeling loving and tender toward yourself? This has a more positive connotation, and it would naturally lead to feeling sorry for yourself too—just as you'd feel sorry for any person you loved who had cancer.

When you have cancer, there are countless valid reasons for your own sorrow. When you suffer the loss or diminishment of something you cherish, the natural emotion that occurs is sorrow. It's wonderful to be in good health, and many wonderful things flow from that—the activities you love, cherished roles in the lives of others, being a productive person, having a future to look forward to. Much of this can be jeopardized or lost because of cancer. It is also painful when the people you love are hurting inside, hurting terribly because of what is happening to you. Of course you want to take their pain away, if only you could. This is another valid piece of your own sorrow.

Everyone, I believe, is carrying some emotional pain. It can go way back to things that happened when we were young, and there can be a thread of deep hurt that is woven into our life story. Often this pain is carried in a sealed-off part of ourselves. And often it is having cancer that taps into this pain and reveals this part of the self that has been hurting for years. This hurt can stem from a precious sensitivity in your nature—a sensitivity that makes you feel certain things, and remember certain things, that are linked symbolically to your current illness.

I have worked with many families wherein a family member had cancer. I look at this family and see the sorrow in everyone's eyes. I ask myself: What can happen within this family that will bring some comfort? Your family is also hurting, so I can pose this question to you. What do you think can help? Maybe your answer is, "Nothing, nothing can help, not really." You might tell me, "The pain we have—it is what it is, we just have to live with it."

Let's see if that's true. Your sorrow has a history. Earlier in life, when you were sad, did anyone comfort you? Was your sorrow known and seen as valid, and did the right person convey that, put his or her arm around you, sit quietly with you, perhaps hold you? If so, then you know what comfort feels like. It did not take your sorrow away, but it hurt less. If you cried, you probably felt better.

If something like this happened to you, perhaps long ago when you were young, then you know the *formula for comfort*: making your sorrow known to yourself and others, having others validate it, having physical contact, crying if you need to. It is comforting to know that you are not alone, that your sorrow is shared, and that others are not threatened by it.

Some people don't know this formula, or what comfort feels like, because they have never experienced it. If this applies to you, you'd probably feel stuck with your sorrow and find ways of dealing with it on your own. But consider this: even though this thing called comfort is alien to you, because it wasn't part of your upbringing, it could still be there *now*, waiting for you, waiting for you to disclose your sorrow so your loved ones could comfort you *now*.

Everyone in your family is already sad, and no one wants to make matters worse. Perhaps your family adheres to an unspoken agreement: *we are not talking about how we really feel because that will just make us more sad.* The premise behind this agreement could be wrong. Maybe the sharing of sorrow within your family would not in fact make family members (yourself included) feel worse. Instead, it might make everyone feel closer to each other. Suppose you end up crying together. I doubt you would say afterward that you wished this had never happened. Your family's sorrow is based on the love you share. Often this love is deepened when a family cries together over a life-threatening illness. It's another reason that people seldom regret these tender, poignant moments, even if they are also painful.

Family Guilt

It is common to feel guilty over all the ways your illness affects your family. It causes a mountain of emotional upset and major disruptions in family life. The family's future may have to be put on hold. You don't want to burden them with your need for care. Of course you feel bad about all this, but why feel guilty? You know it is not your fault for getting cancer. No one blames you, and there is little you can do to spare your family from the consequences of your illness. Nonetheless, you may feel guilty, *as if* you were responsible. Many people with cancer have told me: "It makes no sense, but I feel terribly guilty."

What is the basis for this sense of guilt? As I mentioned in "Cancer and Your Life Story," there can be a religious or cultural basis for feeling guilty. The Bible teaches that illness is caused by sin, whereas living righteously brings good fortune. These ideas have seeped into our culture in very subtle ways, and our culture influences how we think about illness. When things are going well for us in life—good job, good relationships, good health—we tend to assume we are doing something right, living on the right track. In other words, our basic righteousness makes us worthy of our good fortune. There's a flip side to this: if misfortune comes along—such as cancer—it must mean that we were not so deserving after all. This is why cancer can imply something bad about the person who has it. Maybe the person had bad health habits, too much stress, a cancer-prone personality, a character defect of some kind—we are not sure what it is, but it's something, something that creates a stigma around cancer. It can make you feel ashamed or imply that you are responsible in some way. And if you feel responsible because of cultural or religious influences, then it makes sense to also feel guilty.

Feeling guilty comes from the effect of your illness on others, whereas feeling ashamed has to do with your feelings about yourself. There can be a sense of shame that comes with cancer. Again, this comes from what cancer *implies* about you—implications about your character or spiritual health.

You may also feel guilty if your cancer gets worse—and here, again, this makes sense in certain respects. There is a myth floating around in our popular culture, a myth stemming from certain New Age concepts, that if you deal with your illness in the right ways, then you will get better. This requires getting the right medical treatments, participating (if necessary) in the right clinical trials, adhering to the right alternative therapies, making the right changes in your lifestyle and health habits, coping with the stress of your illness in the right ways, maintaining the right attitudes and a strong will to live, practicing the right kind of meditation, getting the right kind of support . . . on and on it goes, bolstered by what you read and what you are told by well-meaning relatives and friends. The basic message is that it's up to you to do the right things, and then you will recover. This is an awful burden on people with cancer. It implies that if your cancer progresses, you are to blame because you failed to do something right.

There is a certain American quality to this myth. It is the American way to be the masters of our own fate. We like to be in control, even in control of nature. With a can-do spirit and the right technology, we can overcome any challenge. We hate the vulnerability and helplessness that are part of the human condition, so we tend to deny these inconvenient facts of life. If someone else gets cancer, it's reassuring to believe that it must be their fault in some way. Believing that makes *us* feel less vulnerable. When someone dies of cancer, it is reassuring to believe that he or she, or a member of his or her support team, must have dropped the ball and failed to do the "right" things that could have prevented or forestalled their death.

Your sense of guilt can be reinforced when family members convey—in certain offhand comments or their body language—their feelings of annoyance or of being burdened by your needs.

Suppose you are lying in bed, feeling slammed by chemotherapy, and you ask your spouse to bring you a cup of tea. You then hear a sigh—a sigh that conveys a sense of annoyance at having to wait on you. This kind of thing can feed your guilt—even if your outward response in that moment is anger or assertion of your legitimate needs.

Your family members can also feel guilty over their resentment toward you. They probably don't blame you for having cancer, but they could resent all the ways it affects them and disrupts their lives and plans. Resenting your illness is not far removed from resenting *you*, the person with cancer. They know they should not resent you and may feel guilty about it, or perhaps they can't even admit it to themselves. They may try to hide it, but it will probably slip out in unguarded moments, and you will notice it.

These feelings that exist in you (guilt or shame) and the feelings that exist in your loved ones (resentment and the resulting guilt) are feelings that can contaminate your most cherished relationships precisely when you need those relationships to be open, close, pure, and filled with mutual love and compassion. If you feel guilty about imposing on your loved ones, you could try to impose on them less—and in the process, deny your true needs for support. If you feel guilty about upsetting them with scary news, you could keep this news from them or try to put a positive spin on it—and in the process, deprive yourself of the emotional outlet and support you need. It is far better for these feelings of guilt, and for the restraints they impose on you, to be openly discussed with your family. Just tell them flat out—that you feel guilty and thus hold back from sharing upsetting news and upsetting emotions. See what they say to that. I suspect the resulting talk will be helpful to everyone.

I am thinking about Larry, a man in his fifties who had an inoperable brain tumor. His left side was almost completely paralyzed. He needed his wife's help with many basic activities and felt terribly guilty about the burden on her. One day he tried to get from his bed to his wheelchair without asking for her help. He fell and hit his head on the nightstand. His wife rushed in; she saw the abrasion on his forehead but could also see that he was not seriously hurt, and she was angry that he had not asked for her help. Sitting there on the floor, his eyes filled with tears as he explained that he hated imposing on her for every little thing and that he feared she'd come to resent him. This was the first time he had admitted how guilty he felt. To her credit, she did not deny the difficulty this imposed on her. But she said that more than feeling burdened by his needs, she felt a deep love and tenderness toward him. She said she liked being able to help, because she felt so helpless about the bigger issue of his terminal cancer. Now she was crying too as she helped him off the floor and into his wheelchair. This poignant moment of shared revelations helped clear the air and deepened the closeness between them.

It can be good to realize that your sense of guilt over the impact of your illness on your loved ones reveals your caring and loving nature. If you felt entitled to unwavering care and attention, then you would not feel guilty to see your loved ones bending over backward to attend to your needs. Although there are no *valid* reasons for your guilt, it may help to see that it stems from your love for your family.

What to Tell Your Children

This final section is addressed to those of you who are parents or grandparents (or even adult siblings) of young children. At some point, you will need to discuss your illness with them, and this brings a special challenge because certain questions must be handled with caution and sensitivity. When I speak of *children* here I am thinking of those younger than age fifteen, although there are no hard-and-fast rules about the age at which young people become better able to comprehend and handle a loved one's cancer. Much of what follows could also apply to an older teenager; you can be the best judge of that.

Here are the questions I want to address:

- What should you tell your children (or grandchildren) about your illness?
- How might you best handle the difficult issue of what to say about the possibility that you could die?
- How should the timing of these disclosures be handled?
- How can you best help them in coping with and adjusting to the disturbing information you'll be giving them?

Of course, no one knows your children as well as you do, and no one, myself included, can presume to tell you how best to handle these delicate issues. Instead, I want to spell out some *principles of disclosure* that have proven helpful to parents and children in my experience and in research in the field. You and other adults in your family can determine, together, how to apply these principles to your children and your unique situation.

Include Your Children

Parents often make the mistake of being overly protective of their children. Thus, to avoid upsetting them, the parents tell them very little, if anything, about the diagnosis and its implications. Children can sense anxiety, however. If no one is telling them the reason for it, they can conclude that it must be too disturbing for them to handle. This makes them *more* anxious. They also pick up on the family rule (the worrisome thing, whatever it is, is not to be discussed) and obey this rule by not asking questions. They end up feeling excluded from what is happening in the family.

Conversely, when you talk with your children about your diagnosis, you immediately send the message that it is not too disturbing for them to handle. This will probably reassure them and reduce their anxiety. They will also feel included. It's a family problem, and they are part of the family. This is very important to children. They will sense that the love and support in the family will help them deal with whatever happens.

Gradual Disclosure

In general, it is better to give children a little bit of information at a time instead of sitting them down and trying to explain everything at once. This gives your children time to adjust to the information you've given, and it could help prepare them for the next piece of information coming their way. You can figure out how much information to share at a particular time by asking questions. Don't assume you know what your child is thinking; find out! For example, you might start this way:

- Have you noticed that Mommy and Daddy seem sad or worried lately? What have you been thinking about that?
- You know I've been going to the doctor a lot. Do you know why?
- Have you ever heard of cancer? What do you know about it?

Open-ended questions like these invite children to reveal their concerns. Such questions convey that it's okay to talk about the worrisome things they have probably noticed, and that it's good to get things out in the open instead of having secrets in the family. If your children answer your questions with a shrug or "I don't know," you might respond with, "Maybe you have been trying not to think about these things. Let's think about them now and talk about it a little." Try to get the conversation started, always asking open-ended questions about what your children think or feel. Most children, once they get the message that it's okay and safe to talk about these things, will begin to open up.

Keep in mind that most children do not want their parents to be worried about *them* at a time when the parents are already dealing with something like cancer. Thus they may deny their own emotions and claim that they are just fine, thank you. Instead of inquiring about their emotions (which they could deny), try addressing their concerns matter-of-factly without conveying you are worried about them. You might say, "It's okay to be worried about this cancer thing. I mean, we are worried about it too, but not so much that we can't pay attention to your feelings or needs."

With young children, it can be good to start with some basic information about the cells that make up our bodies. This will show you respect their intelligence and want them to understand. For example, you might say if they were to look at their skin under a microscope they would see hundreds of tiny skin cells right next to each other. You could explain that each cell knows how to divide in two, making a copy of itself, and they keep doing this until the body has all the skin it needs. These cells know when to stop dividing so we don't have extra skin. You could say that our stomachs (like everything in our bodies) are also made of cells, and that they know when to stop dividing so our stomachs don't get too big. Your children will then be better equipped to understand what comes next.

The next bit of information is about cancer. You can explain that sometimes our cells don't know when to stop dividing, and when this happens, it's called cancer. These cells make a lump, a lump that can get bigger and bigger because the cells can't stop dividing. Then explain that cancer can be bad because these lumps can make it hard for our bodies to work right. For example, if there is a lump of stomach cells growing in our stomachs, then there may not be enough room for food. Explain that these lumps, if they happen, need to be removed from our bodies or we need to take medicine to slow them down or stop them from growing. Be sure to explain that cancer is not contagious and that it rarely happens to children.

So far you have not told them anything about *your* cancer, but they may sense you are leading up to something. It's good to stop at this point and ask, "Okay, what questions do you have so far?" This is better than saying "Do you have any questions?" which can imply that they should not. They may ask why you are telling them this, indicating their curiosity and readiness to hear more.

Suppose you are a woman with newly diagnosed breast cancer. After explaining the basics to your children, you could tell them you had a lump in your breast that turned out to be cancer. You are worried because the lump has to be removed. This validates what your children probably sense—that you are worried—and conveys that it is okay to talk about it. At this point you can ask what questions they have for you.

Answer Questions, But Carefully

You are starting by giving basic information. After that, wait for their questions and be guided by what they ask. Their questions will tell you what they want to know at this point and what they are ready to hear. Try to answer their questions simply and directly, in terms they can understand.

I advise that you refer to a lump or tumor honestly as "cancer." Yes, this can be a delicate matter. Your children have probably heard of someone who died of cancer. Because you're telling them, in the preceding example, about your breast cancer, it would be understandable for them to conclude that *you might die*. They may not be ready to ask about that, but I have found that it's good to address this worry even though they are not voicing it. You might say, "You have probably heard of cancer and that people can die of it. But most of the time people do not die of it. I just wanted you to know that."

You may object that this could create worrisome ideas for children who had none before. That's a valid concern. I suspect, however, that these worrisome ideas are already there.

Suppose your children are precocious and brave and ask whether you could die. That would convey their readiness to hear the answer (otherwise they would not have asked), even though they are hoping, of course, for reassurance. You might say something like this: "Well, that's a very brave question, and I want to give the most honest answer I can right now, which is that we don't know. It depends on how bad it is, and whether the medicine I take for it works. But I think I will be okay. And you should know this too: We are going to do everything possible to make the cancer go away. We are going to the very best doctors. We will be taking care of all that." This last point is to reassure them that the adults in their life are on top of this. It's an adult problem and will be handled by adults. They do not need to worry about that. You might also add that you will tell them as soon as you know more about it. This respects their desire to know what is going on.

Consistency

Whatever you tell your children about your illness, it should be consistent or congruent with what they observe. Sometimes parents downplay the seriousness of the cancer when talking to their children, yet the children observe that the adults in the family are more worried or upset than would make sense, given what they had been told. Thus they would assume the problem is more serious, but they are not supposed to know about it. As I said earlier, this will only increase their anxiety.

Nip Guilt in the Bud

Young children tend to assume that whatever happens in their world has something to do with them. They think in egocentric and omnipotent ways. This phenomenon has been observed in children whose parents are getting divorced, and it can also occur if a parent becomes ill. Suppose the child has been angry at the parent, and soon thereafter learns this parent has cancer. The child could believe that their anger caused the parent to get sick. Or suppose the parent had been angry at the child, perhaps for telling a lie. The child could believe that the parent's anger made the parent sick, or that they did not deserve healthy parents because they had been bad. Young children can't easily articulate these troublesome beliefs. In many cases such beliefs are unconscious—the child is not even aware of them.

If you have young children, there is no reliable way of knowing whether they blame themselves for your illness. So it's good to reassure them that your cancer has nothing to do with anything they ever thought, felt, wished, or did. You might also say that your cancer had nothing to do with *your* being angry or sad about anything they've done.

Children who have lost a parent to cancer or some other illness can believe that the parent died because he or she did not love them enough. Thus they could feel angry at this parent, but they could also feel guilty for not being lovable enough to make the parent want to get better. They know other children whose parents are healthy. Why did their mother or father get sick and die? Does this mean they were not as deserving as these other children? To counteract this, reassure them there is no limit to how much they are loved and that the parent who died wanted more than anything in the world to get better.

If Necessary, Prepare Them for Your Death

This is certainly the most heart-wrenching part, if it comes to that. How can any mother possibly tell her children that she is going to die? How can any father tell them this? Many parents find it nearly impossible, so they avoid the topic until it is absolutely necessary to discuss. They rationalize that it would be cruel and unnecessary to tell the children while there is still hope.

However, most children, I feel, can adjust to even the most traumatic situations if they are given the time and support to do so. This is why it is important to keep them informed over the course of your illness, which could span months or years. Thus they will not be forced to deal with your death all of a sudden, out of the blue. As your illness progresses, and as you talk to them about what's happening and the *possibility* of your death, they will have time to adjust to this possibility. Thus they will be somewhat prepared for this most awful news, if it should come, because of what you have told them beforehand.

Children can relate to your being sick, because they have been sick themselves. They know what sickness is. But what do they know about death, and how can they understand what causes death, or what death means? Children who are fairly young (even by age four) know that living creatures can die— that life goes out of them and they become lifeless. But that does not mean they know fully what death is or can grasp the finality of it.

What you tell them about death will depend on your religious or spiritual beliefs. You might talk with them about your spirit or soul and where you believe that will go when you die.

It is reassuring for children to think that after you die you will continue to exist in some form and will no longer be suffering. I know of one terminally ill parent who told her young daughter that there is a life force that gives life to every living being, and that after her death, her spirit would go back into that life force and then give life to other creatures being born. A father told his young son that when his mother died, she would be a star in the night sky. After she died, he looked for a star, a star that would be his mother, and found one (it was the North Star) that was shining bright. These concepts can be helpful to children. They still have to deal with the loss of a parent, and with missing that parent, but it comforts them to think that the parent who died is somewhere else and no longer in pain.

It can be a mistake, I think, to tell a child that God wanted a parent to be with Him in heaven. This can make the child angry at God. It also conveys, in so many words, that God's desire is more important than the child's need for a parent. This could make the child feel his or her needs do not count for much. Children who internalize such a message will not be inclined to know or value their own needs and the importance of honoring them.

No matter what religious or spiritual beliefs you share with your children, it can also be helpful to explain how happy and grateful you are that you got to live, and that you got to have children who have been a joy, and that your heart is filled with gratitude even though you must die before seeing them grow up. By doing this, you can impart a precious lesson to your children—the lesson that gratitude for what they have can comfort them in times of pain and loss. In dealing with your death, part of their sorrow is sorrow for you (for having to die) in addition to sorrow over their own loss. Their sorrow for you can be softened a bit if they know you feel happy about your life and grateful for them.

Often children have very practical concerns they do not feel comfortable asking about. For example, they may worry (if you should die) about where they will live and go to school and who will take care of them. You can give them some reassuring information about all this, even if they do not ask.

Your Children's Future

This principle is related to talking with your child about your eventual death, if that becomes inevitable. Children can feel guilty about getting to live when you have to die. This is called *survivor guilt*, and it can cause children to become depressed, listless, lifeless. This can be their way of being close to you—of identifying with you—in death. To counter this, it's important to admonish them that their job is to go forward with their own life and make it a life full of joy and success. You can explain that you would be very unhappy if their love for you, or feeling sorry for you, prevented them from doing that. You might say: "Just because I have to die, that does not mean that you can't have a long and joyful life. You must give yourself permission to do that." Tell them that this is your dying wish for them and that they will honor you by heeding this wish.

I know a man who gave his ten-year-old daughter a silver heart-shaped locket before he died. When she opened it, there was a little photo of him on one side and a photo of her on the other. He said something like this: "I want you to know I will always be with you in your heart, just as I am with you in this locket. I will be there to love and encourage you no matter what. You see how I am smiling in this photo? That's because I am happy when I think about the long and happy life ahead for you. Whenever you are feeling down, I hope you will open this locket and see me there smiling at you, with love and confidence that you'll be fine." He asked that she wear this locket whenever she wanted and to keep it in a safe place. I saw her at his memorial service, and she was wearing the locket he told me about. She showed it to me, not knowing I already knew about it. She seemed full of confidence that she was going to be okay.

Don't Go It Alone

It goes without saying that there are many delicate and sensitive issues involved in deciding what to tell your children about your illness. Before taking on this difficult task, it is important to discuss these issues with your partner and/or other family members and friends. Brainstorm with them. Do not expect of yourself that you alone must figure this out. They can help you decide what to say and not say. They know your children too, and often they can offer a helpful perspective or suggestion.

After discussing these issues with your loved ones, talk with your children and see how it goes, consulting with your support network if problems arise. Your children, for example, might ask a question that really throws you, and you don't know how to respond. It's okay to say you need to think about their question and talk to them later. In the meantime, you can see what others have to say about the matter.

If you are married or in a committed lifetime relationship, it is important that both of you discuss these issues beforehand and make sure you are on the same page. Because your children belong to both of you, your life partner has a right to participate with you in deciding what to tell them or not tell them. Your children might want more information than you are giving but not feel comfortable asking you. They might go to your partner with these questions. Ideally, your partner will know what to say because the two of you have already discussed these issues and reached an agreement about how to handle such questions.

The people in your support network are also there to support your children. If they know what you are going to be telling your children, they can be there to help the children afterward by checking in with them, seeing what questions or worries they have, and reassuring them that they are not alone.

One final word of advice: All of these issues are obviously touchy and complicated. Handle them as best you can—and do not expect to handle them *perfectly*. No one could do that. There are too many unknown variables involved. For example, no one can read their children's minds and thus know exactly what they need to hear or not hear at any given moment. The manner in which you (and your partner and support network) handle these matters is a work in progress. You will make adjustments as you go, depending on how your children react to what you tell them. There is no way to make it easy for your children to deal with your illness or (if this becomes necessary) to deal with your death. The best you can do is to make it a little easier for them.

THREE

Learning from Your Emotions

Robert was diagnosed with lung cancer at age fifty-eight. The tumor was removed and there was no indication it had spread. He had six months of chemotherapy and periodic checkups after that. Two years later it showed up in his brain. No other metastases were found, and the brain tumor was operable. He was scheduled for surgery on May 17. His son, Devon, was a senior at Brown University. His wife asked Robert if he'd like Devon to come home when he had surgery. Robert said no. Devon was getting ready for final exams and working on his senior thesis. Robert didn't want him to fly home to San Francisco at such a difficult time. There was more to it, however. Robert did not feel he and Devon were particularly close, and he blamed himself for that. Robert had seldom been home when Devon was growing up. He had worked long hours and weekends running a small construction company that he owned. He sought to make enough money so Devon and his sisters could attend top-notch schools. He told me it was ironic that he worked hard for the sake of his family, but being close to his children had suffered in the process. He said he felt fine about Devon staying at school instead of coming home for his surgery. I asked him whether Devon might want to be there nonetheless. "I don't think so," he said, "not for this, not at this time." He added: "I mean, if I was dying or something, I'm sure he'd come home then."

On May 17, when Robert was about to go into surgery, Devon showed up at the hospital. He was carrying an old baseball glove, a gift from his father when he was ten. He had saved this glove, he told his father, because they were finally going to find time to hit some balls and play catch after his surgery. He put the glove on his father's chest as they wheeled him away. He told him to hold it there during surgery as a reminder that Devon would be waiting, ready to play with him as soon as he was back on his feet. Robert was sobbing all the way down the corridor to the operating room. After the surgery, when he woke up in the recovery room, Devon was there with his mother and sisters. Again, Robert wept.

We could talk about what Robert felt and about all the factors that contributed to his emotional response. But let's focus on this question: What did Robert *learn* from his emotions?

Martha Nussbaum, a philosopher at the University of Chicago, has written a magnificent book on emotions called *Upheavals of Thought: The Intelligence of Emotions*. She makes the point that our emotions reveal what is important to us and how we are sizing up our current situation in relation to that important thing. Here's a quick example: You probably felt scared when you learned of your cancer diagnosis. Your fear showed that you valued your life *and* that you regarded your diagnosis as a threat to that life. Our emotions also have a history, and this history imbues our emotions with personal meaning. Your fear of cancer is related to other threats you have faced in your past, and this history gives your fear a nuance of meaning that is distinctly yours. Other people can put themselves in your shoes and know what it is like to feel scared. But this is not the same as knowing *your* fear. Your fear of cancer is personal to you. It is about everything you might lose, and only you know that. The same is true for your hope. Other people can know what it means to have hope. But *your* feeling of hope is about everything your future life means to you.

Our emotions teach us what they mean—about ourselves, what we value, how they link to our personal history, and our appraisal of our situation and the significant people involved. I will give three case studies later in this essay to illustrate this point. For now, however, let's get back to Robert.

Robert had said, in effect, that it was not important to him for Devon to come home for his surgery. Moreover, he did not think Devon would *want* to come home; in other words, he underestimated how much he meant to Devon. Robert's emotional response to Devon in the hospital indicated that it *was* important to him for Devon to be there, and it touched him that Devon wanted to be there. His emotion taught him something essential and powerful about his closeness to his son. It also brought to the surface an underlying sorrow over all the missed opportunities to be a father for Devon when he was young, a sorrow that spoke volumes about what was emotionally important to Robert—namely, to be close to his children.

There was an additional factor that entered in. Robert had said he would want Devon to come home if he was dying. When lung cancer spreads to the brain, it suggests a very poor prognosis (even if the brain tumor is operable). On some level, I believe, Robert knew this, even though he voiced optimism that the brain surgery would take care of the problem. When Devon showed up at the hospital, it signaled to Robert that Devon knew the awful truth about the meaning of the brain tumor. Otherwise Robert might have said: "Why are you here? I'm just having surgery, and I'll be fine." Instead he broke down with emotion. He apprehended the meaning of Devon's being there—namely, that time was short and he wanted to be close before it was too late.

The point of this example, and the point of this essay, is that there is much to be learned from our emotions. They can teach us things we don't know on a conscious level. As the seventeenth-century romantic philosopher Blaise Pascal put it: "The heart has reasons that our reason does not know." When we pay close attention to what our emotions are teaching us, we can better understand what's behind them. Knowing our emotions is one way of knowing ourselves.

While reading the following case studies, try to think about *your* emotions and what they might be teaching you. Some of you might object that your emotions are pretty straightforward and the reasons for them are plain for anyone to see. This is partly correct, I think. There is a surface level to our emotions; they are what they are, and on that level they are not very complicated. But at a deeper level our emotions are complex, not just because of the possible meanings behind them (as in Robert's case), but because they are influenced by many different factors that are seldom perfectly consistent. It is common, therefore, to have mixed emotions about something. Your emotions in response to cancer are also influenced by many different thoughts—thoughts about the future course of your illness, your ability to cope with the challenges it presents, the capacity and willingness of others to help you, and what others expect of you. Most likely, you have mixed thoughts about these matters, and thus mixed emotions about them.

Exploring and coming to understand your emotions can enable you to communicate them more fully, with the subtleties of meaning of what your personal experience is really like or really about. When your loved ones understand what you feel and why you are feeling that way, you will feel less isolated—less emotionally alone, so to speak.

I understand that the prospect of sharing your emotions may rub you the wrong way if, in your experience, this has often led to more trouble. You might believe, for example, that others would be burdened and resentful if you voiced your feelings. Such a belief did not come from nowhere. Perhaps it was true in your past, so you think it would be true *now*. Or you may think that sharing your emotions will cause others to feel sad or worried and that it would be *your job* to make them feel better. Maybe this used to be true, and you ended up feeling responsible. Perhaps now your loved ones only want to care for you, as opposed to expecting you to take care of them. If we consider the emotional implications, we may see that their desire to care for you comes from a deep and abiding love for you (as opposed to feeling a duty or burden that they'd resent), and that sharing your emotions shows that you trust this love, that you love them too, and that you want their understanding and support.

When you see how your past experience is influencing your emotions, you might want to adjust your emotional response so it is more fitting to your current situation. A woman with bladder cancer told me that when she was young her emotions were consistently misunderstood and often judged to be wrong. She therefore assumed that if she shared her emotions now she would be misunderstood and judged. With some trepidation, she launched a trial balloon by alluding to her fear of dying. She was thankful to find that her loved ones were understanding and sought to comfort her, and she became more open and more inclined to reach out for support.

Emotional support doesn't always have to come from the outside. Of course, when we are upset over something that we want others to understand, it is comforting when they do. But even when no one else understands, you can still comfort yourself. This is called self-compassion. It can feel good to feel sorry for yourself. A woman told me she had never cried over her illness until a metastasis was found in her lung. After learning this news, she sat in her car in the parking lot and sobbed. "I was crying so hard I could not drive home," she said. But then she explained that it was comforting. I think she comforted herself by finally validating her own sorrow and having empathy for herself.

The emotions that cancer causes are always individual and personal. They feel a certain way, or have a certain emotional tone, because of what they mean and because of all the thoughts that swirl around inside the emotion in question. Here are some examples.

Diana and Breast Cancer

Diana was diagnosed with breast cancer when she was forty-two. She was happily married but had no children. She had an MBA degree and worked for a marketing firm. More than anything else, her diagnosis made her profoundly sad, and this sadness had some distinctive features that stemmed from her personal history.

To start, her diagnosis felt like a comeuppance because when she was growing up her four siblings had all been jealous of her looks and intelligence. She felt guilty about these positive traits because they made her siblings feel bad about themselves. Although she tried not to flaunt these traits or take advantage of them, she nonetheless thought they enhanced her success in life. She thought her siblings might even be pleased about her diagnosis because it cut her down to size. She hated this thought, but there it was.

Next, she felt she was not supposed to cry, and this contributed greatly to her sorrow. She acted as though it was her job to take care of the emotions of others; she therefore suppressed her own emotions and put up a strong front. This sense of responsibility stemmed from the message conveyed by her father, throughout her childhood, that she should not dress in a cute manner or talk about her good grades because it would make her siblings feel bad. (I don't know whether her father actually said such things, but this was *her* memory and her conclusions.)

It seemed to Diana there was no way she could be comforted. For her, comfort did not seem to exist. This greatly increased her sadness. The more I learned about her history, the more it made sense. All through her childhood, she had felt she could not take pleasure from being pretty or smart. This seemed very unfair to her, and it seemed no one knew and no one cared. No friend or relative gave her a hug and whispered in her ear that they understood; no one was there to comfort her in this way.

Finally, Diana felt sad because she was childless—but it was more complicated than that. Before her diagnosis, she was sad that she had no children; afterward, however, she was relieved that she had no children to leave alone with her husband if she died. "My being a mother, it wasn't meant to be," she said. "It's better this way." But this idea made her feel all the more sad. It's a very sad theory—the idea that she was somehow fated to remain childless and die young.

Diana's sadness was complicated and deepened by all these underlying meanings. It's sad enough to have breast cancer when you are only forty-two. It's all the more sad to think you deserve to be knocked down to size, that you have to bury your true feelings, that you cannot be comforted because no one understands, and that your infertility has turned out to be "for the best." Yet all these thoughts were embedded in her sorrow, woven through it like a tapestry that buried her with its colossal weight. Understanding these influences was the first step to unraveling her personal tapestry of sorrow.

Mark and Malignant Melanoma

Mark was diagnosed with malignant melanoma when he was forty-seven. He first noticed it on his forehead, but he procrastinated and ignored it for two months. He told himself it was just a bad mole and nothing to worry about. He combed his hair over it to hide it from himself and others. He was careful not to look at it. After a few weeks, he finally took a peek. He deceived himself into thinking that it had not changed much (he later admitted it was larger and partly purple, partly black). He gave it more time to heal on its own. He continued his routine of covering it with his hair and not looking at it.

His main fear at that time, he told me later, was that it would have to be removed and leave an ugly scar. He was especially worried that a skin graft might be needed. He said he was not worried about its being cancer.

Mark was thinking of seeing a doctor about it when his partner, Adam, noticed it for the first time. Adam said it looked nasty and should be checked out by a doctor. Mark procrastinated for another few weeks, then made an appointment with his doctor, who said it should be examined by a dermatologist. Mark did not ask questions that could reveal things he didn't want to know. For example, he didn't ask whether it looked serious.

His doctor asked the receptionist to make an appointment for Mark to see a dermatologist as soon as possible. Understandably, this urgency scared Mark. He also felt embarrassed that perhaps the doctor didn't trust him to follow up on his own.

When the dermatologist saw the lesion, he said that it might be melanoma and should be biopsied. Mark knew of someone who had died of melanoma; thus, searching for reassurance, he blurted out: "If it is melanoma, it just has to be removed, right?" It was a brave question, however, and seemed to show the beginning of a new approach. The dermatologist explained that sometimes melanoma is caught early and only needs to be removed, but that tests are always done to see if there is any sign it has spread. Again, Mark asked a brave question, while hoping for reassurance: "Does it look like it was caught early?" he asked. The dermatologist said he could not tell by looking at it whether it was early or not.

The biopsy was positive, and so was a sampling of lymph nodes in his neck. The melanoma on his forehead was removed, along with some surrounding tissue, and a skin graft was needed. He also had a lymph node dissection, during which several nodes in his neck were removed. The scar on his neck was about five inches long. Scans were performed that found no evidence of any other metastases. However, he was told that there was about a 65 percent chance that microscopic metastases had occurred, which would be too small to show up on a scan, and that interferon treatments were warranted to help his immune system combat these metastases if they were present. He was told that only time would tell whether he was cured or not. If there was no recurrence over the next ten years, he'd probably be out of the woods at that point. He would have to live with uncertainty and wait for that long.

First, let's talk about the nuances of meaning in Mark's fear, nuances he became aware of as he delved into what he feared and why he feared it. He blamed himself for his procrastination, and he felt that he was doomed to pay a heavy price for it. He expected to die of melanoma. As we will see, his procrastination was based on vanity, and he regarded his vanity as such a despicable flaw that he did not deserve to live. His vanity led to procrastination, which led to avoidance, which led to a more serious melanoma, which led to feeling doomed. These were all mixed in with his fear.

Mark's vanity had an unseemly history. He took pride in his good looks and dreaded having surgery on his forehead. His partner, Adam, was also good-looking, and this reflected back on Mark in a positive way. In his twenties, Mark had been in a long-term relationship with a less attractive man. Although he had loved this person, he eventually broke off the relationship because he felt embarrassed to be with a man who was less attractive than he was. Looking back, he felt ashamed that he ended the relationship for such a superficial reason. It was all about his vanity, he said. It was why he ended the relationship, it was one main reason for being with Adam, and it was largely why he'd avoided going to his doctor about the bad mole on his forehead. He had already paid a heavy price for his procrastination. It resulted in more extensive surgery, both on his forehead and neck, and thus more cosmetic damage. It was ironic: by seeking to protect his good looks, he had ended up with a greater cosmetic defect. This irony held a certain meaning for him: because he was vain, it was precisely his vanity that was attacked. This cemented the idea in his mind that his vanity was his most serious flaw. "I got myself into a horrible mess," he said. His fear had been infected by guilt over his vanity and his expectation that he would receive the ultimate punishment.

On the other hand, Mark did not let his vanity dictate the course of his medical treatment. Had he acted on his vanity, he would have resisted a wide reexcision of the local area, the lymph node biopsy, the lymph node dissection, and the interferon treatments, which were physically debilitating. These extreme measures were precautionary rather than absolutely necessary. Yet he embraced them, even though they had negative cosmetic and physical consequences. He felt proud that he was taking this approach. He felt that he was correcting a flaw in his character. He saw that he could feel good about himself as a person, independent of his appearance or physical prowess. This was a positive development, and he attributed it to his melanoma diagnosis and the lesson it implied.

Herein lies another nuance of meaning in Mark's fear: it was tempered by genuine hope. He had made positive changes that enabled him to feel deserving of a second chance, deserving of survival. This hope mingled with his fear. It softened it and made it less ominous.

Most people with cancer live with some combination of fear and hope. When you are afraid, does your hope enter in to balance it? And when you are feeling hopeful, is it tempered by your legitimate fear? How you balance these is personal to you, as is the content of your fear and hope. Your fear can teach you about yourself, about what you cherish and why you fear losing that. Mark feared losing his good looks, but he also felt guilty for prizing them so highly. Your hope is partly grounded in feeling worthy; it points to *why* you feel worthy. Mark felt worthy once he overcame his vanity. When you delve into your hope and fear, it will take you to these personal meanings. It can' be good to know them, just as it was in Mark's case.

Claire and Rectal Cancer

Claire was the youngest of two girls. The family lived in Arizona. Her parents divorced when she was two years old. She and her sister continued to live with their mother, but had regular visits from their father. She adored her father. When she was five, her mother and her mother's boyfriend moved to Mexico City, taking Claire and her sister with them. Her mother apparently hated her father and wanted to get away from him. She did not tell him about the move and left no contact information. He did not know where they had gone. Claire could not recall any explanation about the move. "All of a sudden we were in Mexico City and I didn't know if I'd ever see my dad again," she said. From what she told me, it seemed that she was treated as if she had no rights—no rights to an explanation, and no rights to a relationship with her father. She seemed to accept this state of affairs as just the way things were.

When she was six, she entered the first grade in a Spanish-speaking school. She did not speak Spanish, could not understand anything in class, and made no friends. I was taken aback to hear this, which seemed to surprise her. In her mind, it was just the way things were, and she seemed to accept it. Again, it seemed she was treated as if she had no rights—no right to attend a school where she might learn something, and no right to make new friends.

The issue of Claire's rights shed light on her emotional reaction to being diagnosed with rectal cancer at age thirty-eight. The tumor was low in the rectum and could be removed without requiring a colostomy. But it had invaded local lymph nodes, and chemotherapy was warranted. She was told that her long-term prognosis was about fifty-fifty.

When I first met Claire, she was very cheerful and didn't seem upset about her diagnosis. She had been surprised that, while attending a support group, the other group members gave her feedback that she seemed overly upbeat. She therefore wanted to meet with me to make sure there wasn't "something missing" in her reaction. Mostly she felt on top of the world, but she had a nagging feeling that maybe she didn't get it. She was afraid she wasn't fully grasping the seriousness of her illness, and she wanted to "be real," as she put it.

Claire seemed genuinely happy in her marriage and her job. She said she was more happy, before her diagnosis, than she ever thought possible. This happiness persisted even after her diagnosis. I had the good luck of asking her a very relevant question—namely, whether she felt that she had already attained her fair share of happiness in life, and that she'd therefore have nothing to complain about if she were to die. This question really floored her. She said something like, "Oh my God, could that be true?" She thought it was true, but hated to admit it.

Earlier in this essay, I referred to Martha Nussbaum's point that our emotions reveal what is important to us and how we are sizing up our situation in relation to that important thing. Applying this to Claire, she would be upset over her diagnosis if two elements were present: a sense that having more life was important to her *and* a sense that her cancer was a serious threat to that extended life. This second element was definitely present. She readily admitted there was a good chance of her dying of cancer. But this did not seem to matter to her. In other words, the first element was missing. She did not regard her survival as important. I know this seems odd, and it seemed odd to me. But the way she felt about her survival made sense in the context of how she had learned to think about her rights. As a child, she had internalized the idea that her life situation (being separated from her father; going to a Spanish-speaking school) was an acceptable state of affairs, and she therefore accepted it without complaint. *In her mind, the situation that she found herself in set the norm of what she was entitled to.* If she had a right for things to be better, then certain things would not be acceptable. Her mother's actions conveyed to her that she had no such rights. She complied with this message by making these beliefs her own. Thus, with regard to her cancer, if it were to advance to a terminal stage, she would regard that as an acceptable state of affairs. That, in any event, was how she felt.

There is a law in chaos theory that applies to all natural phenomena, and I believe it applies to psychological phenomena as well. The law states that everything in nature has "a sensitive dependence on initial conditions." Initial conditions have a powerful rippling effect in what evolves from them. The initial conditions in our childhood have a power-ful rippling effect on our subsequent psychological develop-ment. Claire was very sensitive to the initial conditions of her childhood—conditions that implied to her that her rights were defined by what she was given or not given. Only a very sensitive child, and a child who wanted desperately to safe-guard her relationship with her mother, would pick up on this implied message and make it her own.

I met with Claire every week for almost two years. During that time, I tried to send her a different message—namely, that she had a right to a life of happiness, an early death would deprive her of that, and she had a right to be upset. Slowly, it seemed that she internalized this message, and as she did, she became more appropriately upset about her cancer. This was an interesting development: usually therapy helps people feel better, but in Claire's case, it made her feel worse. Fortunately, she regarded her emotions as more real, and she was happy to have them because they were based on a better assessment of what she deserved.

If we return now to our theme about the nuances in one's emotions—nuances that are based on one's personal history—we can see that Claire's fear meant something to her that was very personal, and very moving. She said *her fear felt good.* Isn't that remarkable? Usually, we don't like to feel afraid. But in Claire's case, her fear meant she had a right to more life. She wanted to embrace that idea and to hang on to it through thick and thin, even if it resulted in great anguish.

Two years after her diagnosis, she went in for a routine chest X-ray. The technician wanted to take another view because he thought he saw something that was irregular. When he left the room, Claire began to cry. She had never cried before about her cancer. "It scared me," she said, "that maybe it was in my lungs." She added, "It felt good to be afraid and to cry." That is, compared with her initial emotional response to her diagnosis, this response felt more normal, more appropriate—more real.

It also meant her future was important to her, because it represented a period of her life in which good things could happen. Previously, Claire could not recall ever looking forward to something in the future. The future was just blank; she did not see it offering positive experiences or opportunities. But now she was thinking about the future and feeling sad that she might miss out on it. This sadness felt good. It felt good to desire a future and to dread its loss. Everyone who feels sad about their possible untimely death feels this way because they want to live. To this extent, there was nothing unique about Claire's sadness. What was unique to Claire was the good feeling linked to her sadness, a good feeling about embracing her future and all that it held for her. Her sadness was packed with meaning and spoke volumes of how far she had come from the days when she felt perfectly accepting of her possible death because she was happy in the here and now and felt no right to expect more for herself.

Diana, Mark, Claire. Their stories show the impact of one's personal history on the subtle meanings and feeling tone of current emotions. Think about how this applies to you, because your emotions illustrate the same point. Whatever emotions you experience, they have a history, and they carry this history into the present. We do not experience emotions in a historical vacuum. Consider an emotion caused by your illness, and ask yourself: What does this tell me? You might think of it as a door—a door that opens to a long and complex personal history. If you can, challenge yourself to open that door and see where it leads.

To the extent that your own past has been a painful one, following the path of your emotional history could lead back to painful memories and experiences. You might ask, "Why go back and uncover all the garbage back there?" Your past is not garbage; it is part of your life story. If there was a sad or painful chapter in your life, it will color the emotions you have now, in response to your illness. Diana, Mark, and Claire had emotions that were contaminated by their past, as emotions often are. By understanding these connections, their emotions became more fitting or appropriate to their current life situation. This could be true for you as well. Your own emotional history could be a gold mine for you. Dig there and see what you discover.

FOUR

Mastering Anxiety

EVERYONE WHO HAS CANCER has anxiety too, to varying degrees at various times. Often, it's a low-level anxiety in the back of your mind, but it can be there in an annoying, ever-present way. It can keep you from ever feeling totally content. There can be little peace of mind when the future is so uncertain and so worrisome. Anxiety can well up and seize your mind, as if a sleeping tiger had been suddenly stirred. At those times it can seem to permeate your entire being. It can wash over you like a wave, causing an awful, unrelenting dread that you just can't shake. This often occurs as you wait for test results; if the results are good, you can feel the anxiety drain out of you, but not completely. Anxiety can be in your mind but also in your gut. It can be a sickening feeling, like your insides are unsettled and your skin is crawling. You may feel like jumping out of your body, if only you could. Even when others say how well you look, they don't see the inner turmoil. A foreboding has set in and stays with you day in and day out. I have heard people with cancer say that the anxiety is the worst part. Let's talk about this anxiety and what you can do about it.

It may not help to say this, but it's good to be anxious, especially because of what it says about you. It speaks to the things you value dearly, and it shows your courage in facing up to the way these cherished things are threatened by cancer.

Nonetheless, you still hate the feeling, and I don't mean to imply that you should not. Because of the detrimental effect it can have on your day-to-day life, it's good to do what you can to subdue it. Distraction is a common approach. You may even be able to forget about cancer by preoccupying yourself with other things. "I try to stay busy, so I don't think about it." I have heard that many times.

I have also heard, "It does no good to worry about it, so I just take it one day at a time." Is it true that it does no good to worry? You might say that whatever is going to happen is going to happen—that it does not depend on whether you worry about it. It depends on many things, but your anxiety is not one of them. On the other hand, your anxiety can motivate you to do those things that *can* make a difference, such as seeking the best medical care, sticking to difficult medical treatments, pursuing alternative therapies, or improving your overall health.

In general, anxiety puts us on high alert and prepares us to deal with something dangerous in our environment. To avoid being eaten by a saber-toothed tiger, our ancestors needed to be anxious about that when they ventured out into the jungle. Thus our more anxious ancestors were more likely to survive. Ultimately, we inherited the genes that set up the mechanisms for anxiety in our brains. One saber-toothed tiger in your world now is cancer. Of course you are anxious about it and are inclined to fight it or run from it. These responses to anxiety have also evolved. Because of their anxiety, our ancestors went into the jungle with spears and avoided certain dangerous areas. You are in a similar situation with your cancer. You can confront it head-on or try to avoid it in your mind and in your actions. Whatever approach you take, it starts with feeling anxious.

Although your anxiety may motivate you to be proactive in dealing with your illness, it can still feel like an awful curse. In some ways, it's a curse for all of us, stemming from a basic fact of our human existence—that our bodies are vulnerable, and that we must die someday. It's called "existential anxiety"— something none of us can ever fully escape if we are cognizant of this troubling reality. Even those of us who live in denial of death do so to escape this anxiety. Most of us take some solace in thinking that our death is far off in the future, that it need not be confronted now. But it's different for people who have cancer. Death is in your face.

I am saying that it is not bad to be anxious—it is not weak, not futile, not unnecessary—even though the feeling itself can be horrible.

Sometimes, however, people with cancer are more anxious than they should be. I know that sounds presumptuous; I mean, how would I or anyone know how anxious a person *should* be? Consider this example, however. Suppose someone has a very favorable prognosis—a 90 percent chance of being cured, for example—but is *dwelling* on the 10 percent risk, constantly worrying about it, having sleepless nights because of it, and so on. Wouldn't this person's emotional reaction seem out of balance, and wouldn't more optimism be warranted to balance his or her legitimate worries? I would argue—see if you agree—that this person should be less anxious and more optimistic.

There are psychological reasons for being overly anxious. For example, if a person feels guilty about having a favorable prognosis when others do not, he or she may be overly anxious in order to feel less guilty. Or a person could be superstitious and fear that being optimistic would be asking for trouble; that he or she would be punished by cancer for not being more intimidated by it. Such a person would guard against optimism and accentuate being anxious. In the example just given, this person could exaggerate the likelihood of the 10 percent risk— thinking, in effect, that the chances were high that he or she would fall into the 10 percent of patients who die. "It'd be just my luck to be in that 10 percent group," the person might say. Even if your prognosis is favorable, it can still feel like bad luck to get cancer; it can make you feel like an unlucky person for whom more bad luck is in store. For these reasons, a person's *degree* of anxiety would be higher than warranted by the basic facts of his or her medical situation.

Having said all that, let's get back to you and your anxiety, assuming that your anxiety (and the degree to which you experience it) are warranted and that you hate feeling anxious. What can you do about it? I know of four approaches that can help. I learned of these from people who were dealing with cancer. Like you, they hated the anxiety it caused. Here are some ways they sought to master it.

Facing It Head-On

What are you anxious *about*? I know this can seem like a stupid question to someone with cancer. But aren't you anxious about lots of things? It can help to get it all out; make a long list if you need to. Face it head-on. This can diffuse your anxiety of some of its power—specifically, the power to dominate you. Once you name what you fear, once you have the courage to stare it down, you will be less intimidated by it. It's ironic. It may seem that going into your anxiety would only make you more anxious. But it usually doesn't. It makes you feel stronger, and your anxiety seems weaker by comparison.

A man with a brain tumor was given about nine months to live. The thought of dying, he said, filled him with dread. "I can't stand thinking about it," he told me. I suggested that we think about it together. He went first, telling me about the image in his mind of being on his deathbed. Because I knew some of the things he was dreading about the impact his death would have on his family, when it was my turn I mentioned them. We went back and forth for a few minutes. As we did this, the power of his dreadful thoughts to intimidate him faded, and he felt more empowered to look at harsh realities head-on.

When you think about all the things you are anxious about, try to be truthful to yourself and truthful to others. I know someone who wrote it out in her journal and then read it in a family meeting. After reading her journal, there was a heaviness in the room and no one knew what to say. But she felt lighter, having unloaded her fears, and she shared that feeling with her family. It seemed contagious, she told me. Other people lightened up and were even able to laugh at themselves for being so uptight. Her brother actually made a toast: "Here's to facing cancer," he said.

Containment

There is a technique for dealing with anxiety that I learned from people with cancer. I call it the containment technique. *Its purpose is to contain one's anxiety in a limited period of time so it does not take over the whole day.*

Most people find that it works best to do this in the morning. Set aside a few minutes to focus intensely on all the things you are anxious about. Do your best to bring up every anxiety-provoking thought or image you have about your cancer. If new anxieties occur to you during this morning session, so much the better. You want to get it all in front of you, focusing your attention on it and allowing yourself to feel as anxious as you can tolerate. Keep in mind that you are only thinking—you are having thoughts and images, but nothing bad is happening to you right now. You are safe. Even the bad thoughts are not happening to you; because you have called them forth, you are in charge.

After this session, go on with the rest of your day. Here is what will happen: the bad thoughts and images that you had in the morning will come back into your mind. This is what anxiety does; this is how it stays with you. But now you have a weapon against it, a way of putting it away. To the bad thoughts that intrude back into your mind, say sternly and with conviction: "I already thought about you this morning, and I don't need to do it anymore today. I will get back to you tomorrow morning. For now, leave me alone. Be gone." The bad thought in question will go away, but it probably won't stay away. When it comes back, or when some other bad thought comes in, respond the same way. Over time and with practice, these thoughts will intrude on your day less and less.

This technique is based on a very powerful insight: we have the capacity to step outside ourselves and become an observer of our own thoughts, and when we do that, we can seize control over our thoughts instead of our thoughts controlling us. Suppose you are driving along and your mind wanders off and dwells on something worrisome. When you become aware of this, say to yourself: "Oh, there I go again, thinking about that. Let's see, I have been thinking about that for a good five minutes, just driving down this road. Isn't that interesting, how these thoughts just came in and took over my mind. Hey, these are the same old thoughts I had this morning. I will get back to them tomorrow." You see what is happening here? You are observing the thoughts that came into your mind, uninvited and unwelcome, and you are taking control of them. Remember that your thoughts *intrude*. All of a sudden, they are there. They are there for a good reason: our minds are oriented to cope with the external world, and in your world there is cancer. The trick is to catch these thoughts, to notice them before they take over.

This technique recognizes that your anxiety is real and valid and based on what you are thinking. Your anxiety and the thoughts behind it demand a certain attention, because they are based on a threatening reality in your world. It would be wrong to deny them. It would trivialize the meaning of your anxiety if you tried to avoid it or distract yourself from it. The aim is to give your anxiety the attention it deserves, but to do so in a limited period of time.

Anxiety itself is not the enemy, but its intrusive persistence in your daily life most certainly is. That's why this technique can be so helpful. But it seldom works perfectly. When the thoughts and images that cause anxiety break out of their cage and attack your mind, it's good to have another tool at your disposal. Let's move on to that one.

Meditative Techniques

Many people with cancer go through their day armed with meditative techniques to combat intrusive thoughts that cause anxiety. Such techniques are based on the insight that we cannot think about two things simultaneously. As an experiment, pick out a favorite photo of someone you love or a special place or event, a photo infused with positive memories. Now, for five seconds, concentrate on something that makes you very anxious. After five seconds, picture the photo in your mind's eye. When you do that, you are no longer having the thoughts that made you anxious. They are *replaced* with positive thoughts or memories.

Henry had metastatic prostate cancer, which he knew was incurable. Each morning he looked at a cherished photo of his daughter. He had taken the photo himself when she was five years old. She was sitting on the edge of a fountain, holding an ice cream cone, and smiling right at him. He had memorized every detail of this photo. On some mornings he'd just glance at it, but sometimes he lingered for awhile to let it soak in. When he went about his day, the thought of his cancer progressing would come into his mind. But he had a weapon and was well trained. He'd close his eyes and imagine this photo, and be flooded with feelings of joy and gratitude, pushing his anxiety aside.

Another technique involves a concentrated focus on your breathing. If you think about what your body is doing right now, you will notice that it is breathing all on its own. You will notice how your chest or abdomen rises and falls with each inhale and exhale. This is what is happening *now*; your anxiety is caused by what might happen *in the future*. Our bodies reside in the present moment, even though our minds can dash into the future or linger on the past. So when you are feeling anxious, bring your attention back to the here and now and focus only on your breathing. This takes only a few seconds. With practice, this can become an automatic response to anxiety.

The ebb and flow of your breathing is a natural process you can use to your advantage in quieting your anxious mind and fostering inner peace. You might think of it as a ready-made platform that you can piggyback on for this purpose. As you inhale, imagine that you are breathing in peace, a peace that fills every cell in your body. As you exhale, imagine that you are breathing out tension and stress. Sit quietly and watch your body do this for you, over and over again. Watch it breathe in peace and breathe out stress. As you do this, your mind will be preoccupied with what your body is doing, and you will *not* be thinking your anxious thoughts.

Research has shown that you can reduce internal stress and promote a physical state of calmness just by focusing on your breathing. If you practice doing this whenever anxiety hits you, you will be meeting anxiety with its opposite—with a sense of peace and well-being in the here and now.

As an alternative to concentrating on a special photo, some people pick a special, peaceful place from their past. It could be a private hideaway place you had as a child, or perhaps a serene outdoor place you know and love. Imagine being there, soaking in the peace and contentment you experienced in this special place. Once you pick this spot and practice being there, you can travel there in your mind in a split second. It can be your unique refuge, your safe harbor, your sanctuary—a place where the anxieties that come with cancer cannot get to you, not while you are there, not while you are reliving the sense of peace you had there.

Enlisting Support

If you think of your struggle with anxiety as a kind of battle—a battle raging in your mind between your worst fears and the inner calmness that must be strengthened and reinforced to keep those fears in their proper place—then it may go without saying that support is essential to succeeding in this struggle. Think about this for a minute. If this struggle is lonely and private, it will be all the more difficult for you. Anxiety can wear you down. It can keep you awake at night, and it can be there waiting for you in the morning. In your struggle with anxiety, you must have support. You cannot go it alone.

Knowing you are anxious, your loved ones may try to instill hope and a positive attitude. This is a common response. They don't want you to be upset, and frankly, they feel helpless when you are upset, so it's easier on everyone when you are full of hope. By encouraging you in this way, however, they can end up denying or glossing over your legitimate reasons for being anxious. If necessary, I suggest you tell them up front that you are struggling with anxiety, that you have valid reasons for being anxious, and that you need them to honor that.

There is more that can be said, however. You could tell those in your circle of support that you are using techniques for containing and calming your anxiety. You could ask them to read those sections of this essay. Once they know about these techniques, explain that you'd like to call on their help when the need arises. Suppose you are having a bad day, feeling especially anxious and troubled. You tell your spouse, a relative, or a close friend, who could then help you with the containment strategy discussed earlier. They could say, "Okay, let's get all your anxieties out on the table, and let's be specific and morbid if need be. Let's take them on right now to get it over with." Or they might help you to focus on your breathing, perhaps breathing in and out with you, inhaling peace and exhaling stress. When you do this, you are no longer alone, and you are not *on your own* in your struggle. People who love you are at your side, validating your anxiety and helping you subdue it.

It is easier for two people to worry about something than for one person to worry alone. I know a husband who said to his wife one day, a day when she could not shake her anxiety about her breast cancer, that he would take over and worry about it more that day in order to give her a break. She was so touched by this that she broke into tears. But then she smiled and said, "Okay." Her smile conveyed her appreciation and also her relief. She told me later that she worried less that day.

Anxiety must be "carried" by those affected by it. But who is going to do the heavy lifting? If you try to carry it alone, in order to protect others, you will be burdened by the dreadful weight of it. If your loved ones make the common mistake of trying to support you by voicing optimism all the time, then it can seem to you that they are not carrying any of the anxiety and that you are left to carry it by yourself. This too will burden you. If your loved ones convey that they are anxious right along with you, then it lightens your load. In the example above, the husband offered to carry the anxiety and it lightened his wife's load.

If your loved ones say out loud that they share your anxiety, they may worry you'll end up being more anxious, not less. I don't think it works that way. Your level of anxiety stems from the perceived seriousness of your illness, and this is related to how others perceive it. When people regard it as too serious to face, they may avoid it or talk around it, which will likely make you feel alone and more anxious (because you pick up on the reasons for their avoidance—namely, the intimidating seriousness of your cancer). In the example just given, the husband conveyed to his wife that he did not regard her cancer as so ominous or overwhelming that he could not face it or carry the anxiety it caused. Instead of acting intimidated by it, he conveyed that it was not too threatening to handle. This reassured her. She felt less anxious because her appraisal of the threat was influenced by his.

Your cancer is a threat to many things you cherish, including (of course) your life. You have sized up the degree of this threat, and your level of anxiety follows from that. You have also taken stock of your ability to deal with this threat effectively and whether there are people around to help you. These assessments also influence your level of anxiety because they relate to whether you feel helpless—up a creek without a paddle, so to speak. These appraisals—first of the threat and then of your resources to deal with it—can be influenced by the appraisals and reactions of others. If your support network regards your illness in a matter-of-fact way, as something that can be handled, then you will feel less helpless, less intimidated, and less anxious.

FIVE

Giving Attitude to Cancer

IN A SUPPORT GROUP MEETING for people with colorectal cancer, one member caused such a stir that I had to referee the
ensuing debate. It started by her saying she no longer believed
in a positive attitude. She said she was preparing herself for
the worst, period, end of discussion. "And I'm done searching
for clinical trials," she added. Right away someone said, somewhat jokingly, that she was a cancer heretic. Another member
said that being resigned and passive was no way to fight cancer. "It sounds like you're just giving up," he said. I came to her
defense by saying that maybe she was just being realistic and
accepting, and perhaps that served her well, given her situation. Someone else said there was always hope, and that we
should hang onto hope no matter what. Another member said
she was hopeful but, if the truth be known, she was terrified
of dying. "But I am not dwelling on that," she said. She added
that if her cancer got worse, she would deal with it then. In
the meantime, she was trying to make the best of each day.
Another member said he did not know what all the fuss was
about because at the end of the day it was all in God's hands.
He mentioned the saying: Let go and let God. "I'm letting go of
trying to control things, so God can take over," he said.

This was just the beginning of an intense, heartfelt discussion about the pros and cons of different attitudes in dealing with cancer. For example, one member said she had total trust in her physicians and followed their recommendations, no questions asked. But then someone else said their doctors could not be experts on *every* form of cancer and up-to-date on all the latest treatments. There you have it, the pros and cons of a trusting attitude. It's reassuring to have total trust and the outcome could be wonderful, but it could also be naïve and result in something being missed.

Certainly you want to have the right attitude, but who's to say what that is? Even that question can cause a heated debate because it implies there is one "right" attitude. In this essay, I will not argue for or against any one attitude or approach. Instead, I want you to reflect on the attitude you already have and embrace all the ways it serves you well, while also considering possible pitfalls and whether another approach might be better for you. Maybe your attitude is fine but needs to be tweaked a little. You can be the judge of that.

Here is one way of defining what *attitude* means: it's a set of ideas in your mind about cancer and your role or stance in relation to it. Your attitude is important for two main reasons: it influences the emotions you have in response to your illness, and it dictates the actions you take. An attitude of helplessness, for example, will feed depression and passivity. Your attitude is also important, perhaps even critical, because your emotions and actions could make a difference in the course of your illness.

When you were first diagnosed, you probably did not step back and say to yourself: *Let's see, what attitude should I have about this?* Instead, your attitude was already there, ingrained in you, ready at hand, for better or worse. Even now, as you read this, you probably *find yourself* having a certain attitude or approach to your illness. Where did that come from? What gave rise to it in your situation? What does it say about you, your personality, your personal history, what you believe will help or serve you well? It can be helpful, I believe, to reflect on all these questions.

We all have certain strengths and weaknesses, traits that empower us to rise to challenges but also ways in which we are vulnerable, fragile. You had those before you were diagnosed and carried them with you as you learned about your illness and the treatments for it. I suspect that your illness tapped into or activated certain strengths that helped you to meet the challenges of cancer. But consider this: your illness may have also tapped into your personal vulnerabilities and caused you to recoil. See whether you can step back and take a look at how your personal strengths and weaknesses have been activated by your illness. Once you are clear about this, you may be able to go forward, embracing your strengths all the more, while also tackling whatever shortcomings you notice and seeking help with those because, being human, you can feel overwhelmed by cancer.

Before giving some examples of different attitudes, I want to make a final point about what your attitude says about you. Cancer can cause a person to suffer in many different ways. Suffering is always very personal. It happens to a person, and a person is not a blank slate. I suspect you brought to your illness a certain way of relating to this suffering, a way of relating that shapes how you experience your suffering and how you respond to it. I appreciate that this idea—that your suffering is something you relate to—may be new for you. But there is a relationship involved because your suffering happens to you and then you respond to it. An ongoing interplay occurs, back and forth as you live with cancer, an interplay pitting you on one side and your suffering on the other. Having cancer is not the first time you have been sick or have suffered from illness. You have a history with suffering. We all do. This history has given birth to your own personal predisposition to relate to suffering in a certain way, a predisposition that also shapes your attitude about cancer.

Suppose, for example, that you tend to relate to suffering with resignation and thus with sadness. In your past, you probably experienced suffering as something you couldn't do anything about, and no support was available or offered. It may have seemed that the only option was to be resigned. This tendency toward resignation is something you bring to having cancer. Suppose, on the other hand, that you have learned to relate to suffering with a fighting spirit. Your emotional response and behavior will be much different.

I have chosen to discuss five common attitudes employed by people in dealing with cancer. This is not a complete list, and I don't present them in any particular order of importance. As you read these, you'll see which applies to you. I don't believe any one of these attitudes, by itself, fully accounts for any person's approach. Certainly your own attitude may include a little of this and a little of that. As I said before, I hope this discussion helps you to step back and reflect on the *meaning* of your attitude or attitudes—that is, what they say about you, your strengths and weaknesses, your personal history, and how you relate to suffering.

A Stoic Attitude

Many people, especially men in the North American culture, respond to cancer in a (seemingly) unemotional manner. They see their illness as one of the bad things that happen in life and bring to it an inner patience, endurance, and fortitude.

Being stoic can involve the suppression of emotion, but this is not always the case. According to classical stoic philosophy (as taught by Socrates and Seneca, for example), life always brings suffering and adversity, events that naturally cause us to be upset. But we should not make matters worse by *dwelling* on the negative and thus causing ourselves to be *more* upset. We should try to accept suffering as part of life. That's the main philosophical point.

A person with a stoic attitude tends not to be galvanized to mitigate their suffering, turn things around, or beat their cancer. Being philosophical about it, they try to take it in stride, roll with the punches, and keep in mind that many people are far worse off.

If you have a stoic attitude, it is probably not because you're trying to emulate Greek philosophy. Perhaps you learned when you were young that it was best to keep the lid on your emotions. You would not be inclined to show your emotions unless, in your experience, it paid off to do so—unless it relieved your distress and elicited comfort from others.

Many people act stoic for the sake of others. For example, you may deny or downplay your emotional upset, not because you really don't feel upset, but in the hopes of making your loved ones less upset or less worried about you. Sometimes, however, people act stoic for their own sake. That is, their emotions are deep and powerful, and they fear being overwhelmed if they give full vent to them. One person told me: "If I start crying, I don't think I could stop."

Another factor that could feed your stoic approach is a fear of negative judgment by others and even by yourself. Suppose you think that others will regard you as weak, pathetic, or overly self-involved if you show your fears or sadness. You may have good reason for thinking this way, given what's happened in the past or with the people in your current situation. But you could be mistaken too. Some people might actually admire your sensitivity (in being in touch with how you really feel) and your courage in expressing your true emotions. Your own identity could also be a source of negative judgment. If you pride yourself in being strong and taking things in stride, then you could criticize yourself as being weak if you became emotionally upset.

One advantage of being stoic is that you are containing your emotions, keeping them from getting the best of you, and moving on to more practical concerns. A downside is that it could involve the suppression of your true emotions, for the reasons just mentioned, thus denying yourself both the outlet and the support you need.

A Positive Attitude

Most people with cancer try to have a positive attitude about it, and we are certainly encouraged to do so in what we read and what we are told. Let's consider what a positive attitude really means.

In truth, it means different things to different people. For some, it means being optimistic and inspired by hope. This can be of immense importance. How could a person possibly endure the harsh medical treatments that are currently the prevailing choices for cancer if he or she did not embrace them with a sense of optimism and hope? I know some people who felt they were just going through the motions and doing what they were told and what was expected, but in their heart of hearts, they were pessimistic about the outcome. For them, chemotherapy was nearly impossible to endure. When the side effects were awful, they'd think: *Why am I bothering with this?* They were more easily pushed over the line toward giving up.

For others, being positive means *focusing on the positive aspects instead of the negative ones.* They may be quite realistic about their chances. But they see real, valid reasons for hope and for being encouraged, and they focus their mind on these. One person told me: "Sure, things could go south, but I push that aside. I can beat this thing. That's my mantra." When she was feeling rotten and crushed by fatigue, her attitude was *Hey, it's strong medicine. It's killing cancer.* That's a positive attitude.

Sometimes optimism and hope can prevent a person from dealing with reality. I admit to a bias here: I believe it is good to face up to things the way they are. I think there is real courage in that. When you do that, you are more likely to do what the reality of your illness demands (such as being proactive in pursuing the best treatments), to get the support you really need, and to be prepared for what could happen. As an extreme case, I know someone who repeatedly said, "It's not over 'til it's over." He refused hospice care and kept searching for clinical trials and alternative treatments in Europe. I saw him in the hospital the day before he died. I could only imagine what he was feeling, and I wanted to offer as much support and comfort as I could. But he said again, "It's not over 'til it's over." (I wondered if he was just trying to protect me by saying that.)

A Fighting Spirit

Although this attitude starts with hope and optimism, it does not end there. Those who approach cancer with a fighting spirit are more proactive in pulling out all the stops to survive. Many of them regard cancer as an invading evil entity that must be fought; they feel personally assaulted and challenged, and they are mobilized with a sense of their own power to prevail over it. One person told me: "Cancer happened to me. Now it's time for me to happen to it."

One advantage to having a fighting spirit is that it motivates you to be an active participant in the recovery process and in treatment decisions, and it helps you to think creatively and consider other options. I know a person with anal cancer that had spread to her lung and liver. She underwent successful radiation treatment for the primary tumor and surgery on her lung and liver. This surgery was partially successful, but she still had one lung tumor and one on her liver. Her doctors were not sure what else to recommend. She pursued some new investigational treatments on her own, and eventually underwent a CyberKnife treatment on the lung tumor and radiofrequency ablation (RFA) on the liver. The RFA was successful, but the tumor on her lung remained. She had heard on the news that Farrah Fawcett had recently died of anal cancer. But this did not deflate or deter her. She sought out a top lung surgeon to take out that last tumor. Her recent scans showed no evidence of cancer anywhere in her body. This is a success story, and I acknowledge that many stories do not end so well, even after the most determined efforts. But in her case, the outcome was favorable because her fighting spirit had compelled her to take action.

Those who have a fighting spirit usually have a certain understanding about cancer—that one's own body fights against it, and that it's a mistake to rely *only* on medical interventions to bring about a cure or forestall the progression of the disease. Your immune system, for example, fights against cancer, and this immunological response can be influenced by your health habits and emotional state. One person told me he was "participating" in his body's fight against cancer by fighting it in his mind and by what he put into his body.

A downside to having a fighting spirit is the enormous burden it places on people to do all the right things in order to survive. This is also a downside to believing in a positive attitude—believing, that is, that it will foster a good outcome. If your cancer gets worse despite all your best efforts—despite your fighting spirit, your optimism, your strong will to live—you may then blame yourself for not fighting hard enough, not being optimistic enough, not having a strong enough will to live.

The Not-Yet Attitude

This is a very common attitude or approach that relates to the life-threatening aspects of cancer, to aspects that can cause a person to feel frightened or depressed. It may not be a denial of these aspects, but it banishes them to a future point in time wherein they may or may not occur. The most common expression of this attitude is: *I will cross that bridge if and when I come to it.* The "it" refers to the progression of their illness that could cause their death. Someone with this attitude might also say, "I am not going to get all worked up and upset over something that may never happen. If it does happen, I will deal with it then."

Clearly this approach is related to having a positive attitude (not dwelling on the negative). But it is different in that it does not necessarily involve a focus on positive aspects. People maintain hope and optimism precisely because they feel threatened *now*, whereas those who adopt the not-yet attitude project this threat into the future, a future that may or may not materialize. In my experience, people with this attitude tend to comply fully with the treatment recommendations but are not particularly proactive in doing anything else.

Their attitude is also somewhat matter-of-fact. It goes like this: "I got cancer, as many people do. I'm undergoing the treatments for it. These treatments may or may not be successful, but of course I am hoping for the best. We will figure out what to do next if the cancer gets worse." I am paraphrasing sentiments and comments I have heard many times.

There is a certain commonsense logic to this approach. That is, we should deal with what is happening here and now, not with what *might* happen in the future. This is especially true when dealing with an unpredictable disease like cancer. It's true that you can get statistics that relate to your prognosis for your type of cancer, but these statistics only give the *odds* of certain outcomes. No one can predict this with certainty.

If you place yourself in this category, I want you to listen to what I have to say, and I will be careful and sensitive in saying it. I think you have this attitude precisely because you *are* worried about the future and believe that the best way of dealing with your fears is to knock the legs out from under them, so to speak, by saying to yourself that nothing bad is happening right now. If you believe this is the best way, it means you have not experienced other approaches that may in fact work better for you. For example, suppose you were to pick someone you could really confide in, someone who would listen with compassion and understanding and make it safe for you to be honest and open. This would be someone who did not need you to be unafraid. Suppose you told this person about your fears and found it good to get those off your chest; suppose, also, that this person said he or she would feel the same way, that you were just being human and real, and that he or she would be there to support you in whatever happened. Suppose, finally, that you found comfort in all of this. You see, your fears about the future are fears that you are having *now*, and thus you need support right now in dealing with them. The best way to get that support is to be open with your current emotions—all of them, however frightening they may feel at first.

A Religious or Spiritual Approach

For many people, their religious faith or spirituality prevails over all other factors in how they think about their illness and respond to it. This may apply to you in whole or in part. I will do my best to articulate the two main elements in this approach.

First, there is the belief that some positive purpose is to be served by one's illness. This positive purpose may not be readily apparent, but those with this belief trust that it is there and will be revealed in due time. Their God (or alternative spirit of power and intelligence that rules the universe) would not allow cancer to happen to them for no good reason. Because of this belief, they seek to subdue their natural response of fear or emotional upset, reactions that get in the way of a more important quest, which is to see the hidden reason behind their illness and be guided by this understanding.

Oftentimes, people of faith see their cancer as punishment for veering off track (being too greedy or materialistic, for example) and as a message or call to return to the precepts of their religion and be closer to God.

I have heard many people cite the story of Jesus in the Garden of Gethsemane before his arrest. It is said that he was in deep anguish and prayed to be spared the bitter cup that awaited him. This was his human response. But then his faith came to the fore and he said, "Not my will, but thy will be done" (Luke 22:42). It is thought that he grasped the reason behind this bitter cup and accepted it. This is the ideal that many Christians seek to emulate, as best they can.

The second aspect of this approach is to believe that the ultimate outcome is in God's hands. Those who share this belief do not feel that it is up to them to control what happens. They participate in the treatment plan, believing that God, their Higher Power, or a force in the universe often works through doctors and medical science to bring healing or relief from suffering. But at the end of the day, if their cancer progresses, they seek to accept that as part of God's plan.

Unfortunately, sometimes the progression of an illness can cause a religious or spiritual person to feel forsaken by God or their Higher Power. When this happens, it can shake the foundations of their faith and add a troubling spiritual dimension to their suffering. In "God and Suffering," I give three case examples to illustrate this problem and suggest a perspective from the philosophy of religion that can help a person with cancer feel less personally forsaken by God.

Now that you've read about these five attitudes, you may be thinking about your own attitude or approach and considering its pros and cons. I hope you will think about this question: what *purposes* does your attitude serve? For example, does it empower you to master the challenges that cancer poses, or does it actually make you more vulnerable or helpless than necessary, perhaps so others will come to your aid? Maybe it prepares you for what might be coming; that could be another purpose behind it. And what do you want your attitude to elicit from your loved ones? Their admiration, their sympathy, their support? And finally, what do you want your attitude to do *for them*? Perhaps to reassure them that you are handling things, to tamp down their fears, to prepare them if things get worse? These are the kinds of purposes that any attitude or approach may serve. If you need to, try to nail down *your* purposes. That will help you embrace the attitude that is right for you.

SIX

Five Existential Dilemmas

1. *Should you know your prognosis?*
2. *Optimism versus realism*
3. *How upset should you be?*
4. *Giving cancer the right amount of attention*
5. *On allowing yourself to be sick*

EVERYONE WITH CANCER KNOWS it poses many intractable dilemmas. These are quandaries that can trouble and perplex you not just once, but again and again throughout your cancer ordeal. I call these dilemmas "existential" in keeping with the spirit of existential philosophy—that is, to grapple with the inescapable and troubling givens in the human condition and to figure out the most fitting human response to them. The dilemmas I am about to discuss are givens, I believe, as part and parcel of your cancer journey, and they are too fundamental to be easily brushed aside. Existential dilemmas are not superficial ones.

I will tackle five of these dilemmas in this essay. My aim is to think them through with you, weigh pros and cons, dissect certain troublesome aspects. I hope this process will help you reach a solution that is right for you. If you have already decided what to do about a dilemma that I take up here, but you are still troubled about your choice, then perhaps my discussion will cause you to reconsider and approach the problem in a way that works better for you.

One approach to the dilemmas discussed here is to analyze them with our rational minds. Our minds are also intuitive and emotional, and wisdom can reside there as well. Sometimes we need to get our rational minds out of the way so our inner wisdom can come forth. The words of seventeenth-century philosopher Blaise Pascal apply here: "The heart has reasons that our reason does not know." Thus a solution to a dilemma can *feel right* even though the rational basis for it may elude us.

Should You Know Your Prognosis?

This dilemma can start right away, when you first learn about your diagnosis and the treatment plan. Like many people, you might assume that the treatment plan will take care of the problem, and perhaps your doctors do not say otherwise. But it is just as common that a key question presents itself—the one about your prognosis—and you feel that you may not want to know the answer, at least not then. If you think the outlook is favorable, then you'd surely want to know. Otherwise you might back away from asking the question.

Doctors often express a cancer prognosis in terms of statistics. These usually state your chances of surviving for five years, assuming you receive the standard treatments for your case. If you make it to the five-year mark, your survival chances after that are usually far better. Sometimes cancer is considered incurable if it has spread beyond its site of origin. In these situations a person's prognosis is often given as an estimate of how long he or she has to live. It's nearly impossible for physicians to be precise about this, so they often give a range; say, six to nine months.

Of course, your prognosis changes as time goes by. If the treatments are especially effective in your case, or if new and better treatments become available, then your prognosis may be better than first thought. If your cancer is treated aggressively, but progresses anyway, your prognosis could be worse. You may or may not want to know about these changes. If you feel that bad news would undermine your hope, you may want to be protected from such news.

When thinking about your prognosis, it is important to keep in mind the nature of statistics. Statistics do not predict what is going to happen; they only state the odds of certain outcomes. Moreover, these odds speak to statistical averages, not to all the cases that are better or worse than average. Suppose a study shows a median survival time of fourteen months when a certain cancer spreads to the liver. A doctor might say the person has about fourteen months to live. But wait a minute. The "median" means that half the patients in the study did not survive fourteen months, *but the other half survived longer*. Some patients probably survived three years and were still alive when the study was published. This fact, of course, provides much more hope than the fourteen-month median. Remember too that statistics are based on the historical track record and do not take into account new treatments that are still in clinical trials.

Statistics can have a devastating emotional impact, but they can also underscore the realistic basis for hope. As an example, let me tell you about Wendy, a forty-two-year-old woman, mother of two, who was diagnosed with stage IV melanoma. She asked about her prognosis and was told she had a 10 percent chance of surviving three years. I feared Wendy would be devastated by this news. At first, she was, and she sobbed in my office. She showed me a photo of her two young children. "I can't leave them," she said, catching her breath for a moment between sobs. "They're just too young, and no one knows them like I do, not even their father." She looked at the photo held cupped in her hand, resting on her lap, and cried some more. Eventually, she regained her composure and said the most startling thing. "That 10 percent," she said, "there's real hope in that. It's one out of ten. I could be one of those." She tapped her finger on the photo, looking down at her children. "These are my reasons . . ." Her voiced cracked and she couldn't quite get the words out, the words to finish that sentence. Finally, in a high-pitched voice that was barely audible, she continued, " . . . my reasons for living, my reasons for fighting, for being one out of ten." She pursued an aggressive treatment regimen, improved her diet, meditated twice a day, went to a yoga class, took Chinese herbs, pulled out all the stops. She joined a support group that I ran for melanoma patients. This was a safe and supportive place to express the crosscurrents in the emotional storm she was living through. Everyone rallied around her. It took two years before there was no longer any evidence of melanoma in her body. It took another year before she could feel that she was cured. She was still doing well when I last saw her, five years after her diagnosis. Wendy would want me to make this point: she did not take credit for surviving. Although she was tenacious in fighting for her life, at the end of the day she felt it was mostly just good luck. She was humble and grateful about it. She was that lucky one out of ten.

What about the point that ignorance is bliss? Many patients have told me that as long as they are pursuing the best medical treatments, they'd rather not know about negative statistics. They want to make the best of the time they have, whether it's months or years or decades. During this time, they don't need to be burdened prematurely with the increased anxiety that their statistical prognosis could bring. They know their cancer could progress and that, at some future point, they may have only a short time to live and get their affairs in order. They will cross that bridge if and when they come to it. In the meantime, they don't want to waste time worrying about something they cannot control.

On the other hand, knowing your prognosis could reinforce the importance of appreciating every day, being close to those you love, pursuing your dreams while you can, and attending to unfinished business. One patient told me: "If I didn't know the statistics, I think I'd become complacent and go back to my old routine." In my essay on cancer as a gift, I discuss the positive changes that a cancer diagnosis can bring. Oftentimes, people are compelled to make these changes precisely because they know their prognosis.

Optimism versus Realism

Let's move on to another common dilemma. Regardless of whether you know your specific prognosis, you know cancer is a life-threatening disease and that there is *some* possibility, even if it's small, of eventually dying of it. Should you be optimistic about your chances, or is it better to be realistic? Perhaps you have bounced back and forth between these two positions. On the optimistic side, you probably focused on all the reasons for hope and embraced the medical treatments in a positive way because they could save your life. Being realistic, however, you'd also think at times about the negative possibilities and dread harsh treatments that might prove futile.

On the realistic side, there is also this frustrating aspect: The "reality" that you are trying to face is inherently vague and undefined. Because nobody knows for sure what this reality is, it can be difficult to be realistic about it.

Ideally, you want to have *the appropriate degree* of optimism and realism (given the statistics that apply in your case) and to reach the best possible balance between these two. That sounds right, perhaps, but it is easier said than done. It is very common for people to *over*react or *under*react to their illness, with either too much fear or too much optimism. As you read what follows, see if this applies to you.

Having Too Much Fear

Suppose you think your cancer is worse than it is, so you have very little optimism about it. You may equate cancer with death, as many people do, and thus *assume* that you will eventually die of it. Or you may feel you are an unlucky person— unlucky because of cancer, and maybe because of previous bad luck as well. Even if the odds were favorable, you could feel doomed to be among the unlucky ones. On the flip side, perhaps you felt (before cancer) that you had been exceptionally lucky, had a charmed life, and had enjoyed more than your fair share of the good things in life. It may seem that cancer balances things out or is a kind of comeuppance. You would not be optimistic that things would go well for you if you feel you've gotten cancer to balance your previous good fortune.

As I discussed in "Mastering Anxiety," sometimes people feel that being optimistic is asking for trouble. It could provoke cancer to teach them a lesson. Thus they accentuate their fears in order to play it safe. This can occur even if your prognosis is favorable. Or, you may feel guilty about that because other people with the same cancer are not so lucky. It seems wrong to celebrate your good fortune (that is, by being optimistic) when others are worse off. Thus you'd be inclined to revert to the opposite of optimism—being more fearful.

Being optimistic is related to feeling *deserving* of a good outcome. You probably don't say to yourself, *I deserve to be cured and am therefore optimistic.* But if you did not feel deserving, you probably would not be optimistic. Do you agree? Feeling no more deserving than anyone else, and realizing that the outcome has nothing to do with what you deserve, could cause you to squelch your optimism and be more fearful.

Having Too Much Optimism

Suppose you are reacting to your illness as if the threat to your life is much lower than it is. A common reason for this reaction is denial, which is a complex phenomenon. It is based on a theory that we unconsciously perceive a threatening reality, anticipate the emotions it would cause if it were conscious, and then block the conscious awareness of this threatening thing. Thus denial is a *defense mechanism* that protects us from threatening emotions. The theory also says we size up our ability to cope with these emotions; if we think the emotions would be overwhelming, we'd be more likely to employ denial to protect ourselves. (It's interesting, however, that what looks like denial could actually be the employment of optimism as a way of dealing with a threat that is not being denied.)

It is not uncommon for people to use denial *initially* when first learning about their illness. There is so much to learn and do during this period. It may not be the right time to deal with all the upsetting emotions. Later, we can let these emotions in. Also, over time people often become more confident of their ability to cope and be resilient and thus feel a bit less threatened by upsetting realities and emotions.

If you believe that a positive attitude is key to surviving cancer, then you may also believe that being realistic, and thus afraid, could jeopardize your recovery. Thus you'd be inclined to suppress your fears and swing in the other direction, having too much optimism.

The Power of Observing Your Thoughts

The point of all this is that it's difficult to have the right balance of optimism and realism because of these various psychological and interpersonal factors that could make you overly fearful or overly optimistic. When this occurs, it can be very helpful to become an *observer* of your thoughts. When you notice you are more fearful than your situation warrants, you can say to yourself, *Oh, there I go again, fearing the worst.* If you notice you have mostly optimistic thoughts, you might say to yourself, *Oh, there I go again, making light of a serious situation.* The first step is to adopt the stance of an observer of what your mind is doing; after that, you can exercise some control. Think of it this way: who is in charge of how you feel—your automatic thoughts, or you?

One final thing to note is that weighing optimism against realism isn't just a judgment call that you make in light of what balance is best for you—it's also a judgment call that your doctors make. Your doctors can help or hinder you in being appropriately optimistic or realistic. Sometimes oncologists cannot bring themselves to be honest about a person's prognosis, potentially distorting the truth by saying there is always hope and more treatments to try. But sometimes they do the opposite and make godlike pronouncements about a person's approaching death. Ideally, your oncologists should have a balanced approach and offer realistic hope while also helping you, if it becomes necessary, to stop fighting and pursue the comfort that hospice care can provide. If you sense that your doctor might be sugarcoating the truth or making dire predictions, it might help to say that you are trying to have a balanced approach and that you want them to take a balanced approach as well.

How Upset Should You Be?

Having too much fear or too much optimism relates to your degree of anxiety. But what about just feeling *upset* (disturbed, sad, bummed out) over your illness? Here's the dilemma: on the one hand, you have every right to be very upset, but on the other hand, millions of people, over the course of human history, have suffered far worse fates, and even right now there are millions of people who would love to be in your shoes instead of their own. Taking that into account, you should not be too upset. Right?

Let's see if we can think this through. The dilemma arises when you place your own situation in a broader context. It can seem the plight of other people should have a bearing on how we feel. There is no objective truth to this; it's really just a thought. Thus we can choose to embrace this thought and therefore moderate our own feelings by considering the fate of others, or we can choose to reject this thought because it deprives us of our own true feelings.

What choice is right for you? The answer depends *partly* on your self-definition or self-concept. One person might say, "I like to be mindful of the fate of others." Another might say, "I like to be in touch with my true feelings and to honor them." To this person, asserting their own emotions could be of primary importance, especially if those emotions have not been regarded as valid or worthy of attention in the past.

Let's think for a minute about how emotions work, and see if that helps us understand how "being upset" fits in. Normally, one's *initial* emotional response to a cancer diagnosis is to be upset. Being upset is based on two elements: your life and well-being are important to you and your loved ones, and you see your diagnosis as a threat to your life and well-being. Given these elements, your initial emotions are totally valid. Later, other thoughts come into play—thoughts such as "Other people have been, or currently are, far worse off, and therefore I should not be quite so upset." This thought is secondary to your initial emotional response and serves to moderate it.

This puts the question in a different light, even though it may not solve the dilemma. The question could be: Should your initial feelings have primary importance, given their obviously valid basis? They come more from your gut and not from your head. Your subsequent emotions are more thoughtful, taking a broader perspective. Maybe those should carry the day. Then again, this broader perspective may serve to make you less upset; that could be the reason for it.

I think a solution to the dilemma can be found in balance. It is not either/or; that is, either you embrace your initial response *or* you suppress that while taking other considerations into account. You can balance the two. You see that you have every right to be upset, but you can balance *your degree of upset* by recognizing the broader context. You would not let this recognition cancel out or invalidate your initial response; nor would you let your initial response hold sway over all other considerations.

The issue of your rights also comes into play—that is, do you have a right to be upset and for your gut emotions to be known and honored? The environment in which we are raised is partly a moral environment about what is right and about whose rights are most important. Here is a little example. Suppose your bike was stolen when you were young, and you went to tell your father, but he was busy fixing something and did not want to be bothered. You could conclude that your right to be upset over your bike was secondary to your father's right not to be bothered when he was in the middle of a project. If such things happened repeatedly, you would develop the belief that your emotions, and your right to have them, were of secondary importance. You would not give your emotions the attention they deserved. You would feel guilty about making your emotions important, because you were supposed to be focused on others.

I have found that many people with cancer are somewhat cut off from their emotions or are reluctant to express them in a manner that does full justice to how they feel. It seems they do not have a good sense of their emotional rights as compared to others. If a man is diagnosed with cancer, but believes that his wife's right to feel safe is more important than his right to feel upset, then he will try to deny his fears or hold back in expressing them. If this man is thinking (unconsciously) that he does not have a right to be upset, he will find himself thinking of other things—such as the worse fate of others—in order to subdue his own emotions. That's why I have stressed the importance of balance. You have a right to feel what you feel. You have a right for this to be known by others, and you have a right to be supported and comforted. You can honor those rights, just as you may also honor your sensitivity to the plight of others who are worse off.

Giving Cancer the Right Amount of Attention

Let's move on to another dilemma: how much attention should you devote to your illness? You are already devoting a certain amount of attention to it, are you not? The question is: Is this the right amount? Many people have told me they are too preoccupied with their illness; others have said they are not giving it the attention it deserves. Can you place yourself in one camp or another?

Let me state the dilemma this way: on the one hand, it's good—in principle—to give your cancer the attention it deserves; on the other hand, it's good not to be preoccupied with it. It's good to keep it in its place so it does not take over your life. The solution to this dilemma, of course, is balance. Let's see how that might work.

What does it mean, really, to give cancer the attention it deserves? We are talking metaphorically here, because cancer does not literally *deserve* anything. The issue, really, is the amount of attention that is *warranted*, given that cancer is a life-threatening disease and not the common cold.

The idea of giving cancer the attention it deserves grows out of a certain way of thinking about cancer. It personalizes it, as if it were an entity that deserves something (lots of attention and lots of fear), and if this something is not given, the entity would be provoked to take punishing action. Of course, cancer does not carry a grudge if you ignore it, and it does not look with favor on you if you pay homage to it by giving it lots of attention. But it can *feel* this way—it can feel that you are asking for trouble if you do not give it the attention it deserves, and it can feel safe (or safer) if you are making it your central, overriding concern.

A patient of mine complained that she was living in fear. We discovered that her fear was actually an unconscious strategy to prevent her cancer from coming back. She was afraid not to be afraid. She came to see that she was thinking about her cancer as an entity that wanted her to live in fear of it. On occasion, she found herself feeling optimistic, and this caused her fear to come right back. Ironically, being afraid made her feel safer. Upon realizing this, she was actually amused! "It's funny," she said. "I complain about being anxious all the time, but if the truth be known, I like being anxious. It's my safe harbor."

When you learned of your diagnosis, you probably reacted with serious concern. That was definitely warranted; a cavalier response would not be. Presumably, you asked serious questions, learned about the pros and cons of different treatments, and decided to pursue the best treatments, all things considered. Now what?

Here is where the issue becomes more complicated, in terms of how much attention to devote to your illness. The maximum amount of attention would be equivalent to a full-time job, with overtime. You would read several books about your type of cancer and become a virtual expert. You would read the medical literature to be up-to-date on the latest research and clinical trials. You might consult with experts in various cancer centers around the country. You would listen to the recommendations of your doctors, but ultimately you would decide which treatments to pursue. For example, you might participate in a clinical trial, even if your oncologist knew little about it. You would also learn about complementary or alternative treatments for your cancer. This would involve more reading, Internet searches, and consulting with practitioners of alternative medicine. You would also learn about the role of diet and nutritional supplements and about the mind-body connections that relate to your illness. You might learn, for example, about the role of meditation and yoga in helping your immune system; you would then practice meditation and enroll in a yoga class. You would also join a support group related to your type of cancer. As I said, it would be a full-time job.

The minimum amount of attention would look like this: you would just do what your doctor recommended, no questions asked, and you would avoid learning anything about your specific case. Your attitude would be, *If there is something I need to know, my doctor will tell me.* You would be obedient but passive. You would try not to think about it or worry about it. You would go on with your life as before and keep your illness in the background. To talk about your illness with family and friends would be to make it important, to pay attention to it; you would do very little of that. I have heard patients say: "I don't want to make a career out of having cancer."

As you can see, we have two extremes here. Obviously, some middle ground is needed. It's a dilemma, however, because no one can say, with godlike authority, what sort of balance is appropriate and warranted. Most of the patients I know have wanted to give cancer its due, but have not wanted it to take over their lives. They have struggled to find the balance that was right for them.

Let's think about why a person might go overboard, in doing too much, and why someone might go to the other extreme, in doing too little. Certain personality factors play a role. If you tend, by disposition, to be proactive and take-charge, then you'd be inclined to go overboard. If you tend to be more passive and compliant, then you'd be inclined to act similarly in response to your illness. Sometimes, when we notice an aspect of our personality, we feel critical toward it because we don't want to be that way. So ask yourself whether your personality is dictating a response to your illness that you'd like to alter. Just because you *tend* to be a certain way does not mean that you *must* be that way in all circumstances.

There are some other psychological factors to consider. If you are making your illness a full-time job, you probably *believe* in this approach—that is, that it maximizes your chances. You may believe that if you relax, it would be tantamount to letting down your guard and making you vulnerable. You may imagine that your cancer is waiting for you to give it an opening, and then it will strike. Your strategy may be to keep cancer at bay by maintaining a full-court press.

Although this strategy can help you feel less vulnerable, it can also wear you out. Suppose, instead, that you tried to be at peace with your vulnerability. This may seem like an odd suggestion, as you hate being vulnerable and you hate the anxiety it creates. But your vulnerability is a fact, isn't it? There's an old saying: *You can run but you can't hide.* You can run from your vulnerability, but there is no hiding from it. You may rationalize that you can reduce your vulnerability by being preoccupied with your illness and pulling out all the stops to deal with it. It might be better to accept your vulnerability as a given, as an inherent aspect of your existential situation, and to maintain hope *in spite of* this basic vulnerability. Instead of trying to rationalize your vulnerability away, you would let it be what it is but not let it terrorize or paralyze you. You would not be ruled by it. You would not let it dictate an all-consuming anxiety or dictate a response to your illness that wears you out and prevents you from enjoying whatever time you have left.

Suppose you are at the other end of the spectrum, paying very little attention to your illness. There are psychological factors to consider here as well, especially certain beliefs (perhaps unconscious) that could be influencing you. In what follows, I want to call attention to such beliefs, because awareness of them could enable you to step back and evaluate their accuracy. When people do this, they often find that the beliefs behind their behavior are not really valid.

One belief could be that it's best to leave well enough alone. If you were to focus on your illness, you reason, that would just create more anxiety, more unanswered questions, more loose strings. Such a belief could cause you to let it be, or to distract yourself from it by focusing on other aspects of your life. This could be a mistaken belief, however. Perhaps you could devote more attention to your illness without its taking over or getting blown out of proportion.

There could be another belief at work here—namely, that paying more attention to your illness would create a kind of emotional overload on you. Perhaps you regard your illness with grave apprehension and fear that you do not have the wherewithal to cope with it. But you may be selling yourself short. Also, you may fear that, if you were to take on your illness, you would not receive the support you need. But you may be selling your loved ones short. You just might find that, given the chance, they will offer you more support than you expect.

Suppose you have a fatalistic attitude and believe your cancer is going to do what it is going to do, regardless of how much attention you pay to it. Why bother, therefore, to focus on it? Certainly you were not *born* with this fatalistic attitude, nor did you invent it out of thin air. Perhaps there was a time when you were more proactive but became demoralized and beaten down. Perhaps you are acting out an identification with a fatalist parent or older sibling. The problem with fatalism, when it comes to cancer, is that there *are* things you can do to potentially influence the outcome. Learning about the best treatments, then sticking with them, is one obvious example. Not going overboard with treatments and exhausting yourself could be another.

On Allowing Yourself to Be Sick

Here's another dilemma: on the one hand, it's good to allow yourself to be sick (exhausted, nauseated, rotten, and so on) when you are feeling that way; on the other hand, it's good to push yourself to get up and get going, to fight back, not to give in to feeling ill. I suspect that you have been confronted with this dilemma, and I suspect that you have tried to resolve it in the second way, by fighting against the awful physical aspects of cancer and cancer treatments.

Let's think about this dilemma. In my opinion, it's good to allow yourself to feel sick when you are in fact feeling that way. I have a certain philosophical bias here—namely, that it's good to accept what is, insofar as it's an inherent or given aspect of your real situation. I believe in being real. If feeling sick is the reality of your situation, then I think it's right to call a spade a spade and let your physical state be what it is. I know this is a bias, and I know it can be challenged. For example, it could be argued that the reality of your situation is not really a given independent of how you think about it. If you have a "poor me" attitude about it, or believe you are stuck with it, you will be more inclined to feel depressed about your physical symptoms and they will feel worse. But if your attitude is *Surely this will pass and my resilience will carry me through*, then you will experience your physical symptoms in a more matter-of-fact way, without an overlay of self-pity, hopelessness, or helplessness.

In response to this argument, I would say that both things are true. In one sense, your physical symptoms *are* a given. You find yourself having them. They have been thrust upon you, and they cause certain emotions. At the same time, the emotions you have in response to your physical ailments result from the *intersection* of real symptoms with your attitude about those symptoms.

I am thinking of a woman who told me the concept of surrender helped her greatly. She had been fighting against her cancer and fighting against all the physical suffering that came with it. She was not winning these battles. Her cancer was getting worse, requiring more aggressive treatments, and she was feeling worse. She was also exhausted. She felt weary, demoralized, and worn down. She then had a kind of awakening, as she put it. She realized that it was okay to surrender to her illness, and to let it be what it was. She did not have to fight against it. The burden was lifted. She could suffer in peace, she said. Isn't that interesting? If we must suffer, isn't better to be at peace with it?

What about the notion that it's good to push yourself to get up and get going, to resist being passive and resigned? Certainly your resilience and sense of empowerment are enormously important. Many patients have told me if they can just get out of bed and get going, they begin to feel better. One man used to take a vigorous walk in the morning. His route took him up a hill from his home, through a neighborhood and then a park, behind a large mall and back to his home. He said it was about two miles. He could do it in forty minutes. But then chemotherapy just wiped him out. There was no way he could muster the energy for his morning walk. He decided, instead, to take the walk at a slower pace rather than give in to his fatigue and stay at home. He started his walk like a turtle, he said. But after a block he felt a little more energy and could pick up the pace. He said the whole loop took almost two hours. But it was invigorating and boosted his spirits. He was not letting his illness impose unnecessary restrictions. It imposed real limitations on the pace of his walk, but he did not let it deprive him of something that was so beneficial to his physical and mental well-being. This is an example of being resilient and having a sense of personal power in the face of illness, while avoiding unrealistic expectations and pushing oneself too hard.

I have come to believe that we all possess a wellspring of inner strength. I have seen it countless times in countless ways. It's ironic that we are often driven to this deep inner place by horrible suffering. So often it is through our suffering that we

discover what we are made of. There is strength in being resilient, and there is strength in accepting the reality of our suffering for what it is, when we have no choice, really. There is
profound strength of character and spirit in both approaches,
and we give meaning to our suffering when we find and embrace
this strength.

Finding Balance

Here's the thing: balance is the key when it comes to facing
all the dilemmas discussed in this essay. But only you can
find the balance that is right for you. The response that is best
for you depends partly on how you have dealt with suffering
in the past. It's good to check in with yourself regarding that
issue. How have you solved dilemmas in your past? What are
you reconsidering now that you've thought more thoroughly
about those reactions? Your illness challenges you to find the
path that works for you. Your path through cancer is a thorny
one, full of dilemmas along the way, but also full of opportunities for you to honor your inner truth and your inner needs.

SEVEN

God and Suffering

WHEN DAVE WAS DIAGNOSED with pancreatic cancer, he prayed that chemotherapy, with God's help, would work against it. He told his pastor about his diagnosis, and Dave's name was added to the list of people the congregation prayed for each Sunday. He also asked everyone in his family to pray for him. "I have lots of prayers going my way," he said, "and I really believe that's going to help." Unfortunately, they did not seem to help. The cancer spread to his liver. Instead of taking medication for the pain, he prayed that God would intervene. He finally resorted to oxycodone. At first, he joked that God must be too busy answering other people's prayers, but after a while he became disillusioned, discouraged, and even bitter. You could see the anguish on his face. He explained that all his life he had tried to be a good Christian and to help those who were less fortunate. It was a cruel irony, he said, that God had forgotten him in his hour of need. Seven months after his diagnosis he was referred to hospice care. He was depressed, but not about dying, he said. He felt abandoned and forsaken. He no longer believed that he would be with God after he died.

It seemed that Sarah's breast cancer had been treated successfully. In keeping with her Jewish faith, she regarded that as a special blessing. But three years later it showed up in her right lung. She did not ask "Why me?" and she did not feel abandoned. She believed that God was still with her. Her rabbi encouraged her to meet God in her suffering. He said that God suffered with her. She thought of the millions of Jews who had perished in the Holocaust, and she felt a kind of kinship with them. She believed that God would help her deal with her illness in positive ways. She said to herself: "Okay, this is part of life. What am I going to do about it?" Being grounded in her faith and her Jewish tradition seemed to genuinely comfort her. But then the cancer spread to her brain, which had been her greatest fear. She had whole-brain radiation therapy and heavy doses of steroids to control the swelling. She became forgetful and disoriented. It was at this point that she said: "I am slipping away. There is no God here. There is nothing left to do but die."

I first met Michelle when she returned from a retreat at a Buddhist meditation center in Northern California. She was undergoing chemotherapy for ovarian cancer, and the side effects were nearly impossible to bear. Buddhism teaches that suffering is created by our desires and aversions. Thus we suffer less when we meet our desires with detachment and our aversions with acceptance. In her daily meditation practice, Michelle sought to let go of her desire for anything (such as her desire to be cured or to be free of nausea and fatigue), to quiet her mind, and to reside in compassion toward the suffering of all sentient beings. The conditions of her bodily existence, however, were gaining the upper hand. When she was in pain, she could not help but be preoccupied with it. It grabbed her attention like a steel trap and would not let go until the pain itself receded. "I'm a Buddhist failure," she told me.

The experiences of Dave, Sarah, and Michelle illustrate how a person's religious faith can become a source of additional suffering when dealing with cancer. Personally, I hate to see this, especially because I know from many others how one's faith can be an abiding source of meaning and peace, as it was for the man whose story follows.

Martin was raised a Catholic but stopped going to church in his late teens. Nonetheless, some of the basic teachings of his upbringing, he told me, had seeped into his inner being, and he still believed in God. He was diagnosed with colon cancer when he was fifty-two. It had already spread to his liver, and his long-term prognosis was poor. His faith helped him to deal with this in a very simple and yet powerful way. Looking back over his life path—which had not been a bed of roses—he saw many examples of God's love and guiding hand. He told me he was counting his blessings and feeling grateful, instead of "pissing and moaning" (his words) over his current situation. In truth, he had periods of depression when he was terribly sick and fearful about his prognosis, but these feelings were significantly offset or balanced by his sense of gratitude. I saw him in the hospital about a month before he died. His oncologist had just been in to give him some bad news about a recent scan. His wife and two daughters were also there, crying softly by his bed. He said something like: "Look how loved I am. This is how I've been blessed."

The reality of suffering is a persistent and troubling challenge in all religious traditions, each of which offers a way of finding comfort. In the Christian tradition, the evil in the world and our individual suffering is part of God's redemptive plan. You might look at *Evil and the God of Justice* by the Anglican bishop and theologian N. T. Wright to learn more. According to Judaism, evil entered the world because of sin and suffering is now part of the human condition. Although God can seem silent and distant, He is nonetheless present with us when we suffer. Rabbi Harold Kushner takes up this issue in his popular book, *When Bad Things Happen to Good People.* Buddhism is primarily concerned with suffering, for this is a central fact for all living creatures. The Buddhist teachings about life, death, and suffering are explained in *The Tibetan Book of Living and Dying* by Tibetan monk and scholar Sogyal Rinpoche. For many people, their faith is rather undefined and incorporates elements from these and other traditions. If this is true for you, each of these books could help to enrich or deepen your faith as you confront the personal suffering that cancer is causing in your life.

I have worked with people with cancer for many years and continue to be impressed and moved by people like Martin, who hold on to a sense of gratitude for their blessings in life. For many people, this gratitude, grounded in faith, is a powerful and transforming sentiment in the face of suffering. I have found that the deistic philosophy about God, which I will explore on the following pages, has proven helpful to many patients who are trying to reconcile their faith with cancer. Deism points to a deeper theological meaning when people who are suffering are able to count their blessings.

I also want to discuss deism because it addresses the problem of evil—that is, if God is all-powerful and all-loving, why does He not intervene to prevent innocent human suffering? This problem is so intractable that an entire area of theology (called *theodicy*) is devoted to it. When your religious faith and personal relationship with God slam into the problem of evil, you can begin to suffer in a spiritual sense. You may, in your darkest moments, cry out to God for help, only to be met with silence and seeming indifference. It's not just perplexing; it can shake the foundations of your faith and trouble your soul. You may feel unworthy of God's help because of past sins or spiritual shortcomings. Or you may conclude that God is allowing you to suffer because something good will come from it—yet whatever this positive purpose may be, it may also seem that it's just not worth it. At the end of the day, you can feel dropped and forgotten instead of safe in God's loving hands. Let's see if deism can help. And let's see if it sheds light on what to pray for as you suffer from cancer.

God's Creative Purpose

Deism is not a specific religion; rather, it is a long tradition in the philosophy of religion about God and His relation to the world.

Deism teaches that God is good, and therefore God's intentions or purpose in the act of creation were good. But although God was *powerful enough* to bring the universe into being, this does not mean (in the deistic view) that God is all-powerful. Consequently, the goodness of His purpose does not mean that only good things will happen in His creation. If you are a parent, certainly your intentions for your children are good, but other factors beyond your control can get in the way. You feel sad and helpless when bad things happen to your children. Deism suggests it is the same for God.

In the deistic view, God designed a universe that had the maximum *potential* for good results. Thus the universe evolved in ways that actualized this potential. But evil was also possible because God could not preordain a world that was only good.

The basis for this deistic teaching is found in the natural world, a world that reveals God's goodness, wisdom, and power, but a world that also contains randomness and disorder, and thus evil and suffering. These point to the limits of God's power.

The seventeenth-century philosopher Leibniz taught that God created the best of all possible worlds. God was good in that sense, but His power was limited by what was possible (Leibniz thought certain physical laws were given and imposed limits on what was possible). Other Enlightenment deists, such as Newton, Voltaire, and Spinoza, saw things differently. In their view, God created the laws of nature, including the laws of physics. They were not given beforehand or preordained in the nature of any possible world. Albert Einstein's notion of God also followed this deistic tradition. "I believe in Spinoza's God," Einstein said, "who reveals himself in the lawful harmony of all that exists." He said that he wanted to know "the mind of God" that informed the harmony and beauty of the universe and its laws.

God and Cancer

Cancer can be seen as one of the bad things that result from the fact that we are biological creatures. This is reflected, for example, when someone with cancer asks "Why *not* me?" The point here is that we are all vulnerable. Where does God fit into this picture?

From a deistic perspective, God did not intend for evolution to give rise to creatures (us) who would be vulnerable to cancer. We might think of creation as an act of divine faith. God believed that His universe would be predominantly good. He set it up that way. But he could not eliminate or rule out the possibility of evil or suffering. Had He been able to rule these out, He would have.

In other words, we live in a universe that is mostly good, but obviously not *only* good. The key point has to do with God's role in such a world. A tension exists in the universe between God's intention of goodness and the possibility for evil. His faith was that the good will outweigh the bad. This is a fundamental truth that informs all of creation.

When you are suffering from cancer, but can nonetheless count your blessings and feel grateful, then you are allowing the good in your life as a whole to outweigh the evil of cancer.

When you do that, you are participating in God's cause—His cause for the universe and his cause for you personally.

Still, there can be a nagging question: When God sees that His creation is often causing untold misery for us—because of disease, war, or natural disasters—why does He not intervene to change things? Even if we grant that God's power is not unlimited, it can still seem that He would have enough power to intervene in this world to eliminate innocent suffering. But consider this: the power to create something does not necessarily mean the creator also has the power to change that thing once it begins to evolve according to natural processes. That's the deistic view. Perhaps this analogy can help: Suppose we regard an acorn as created by God, but once it has been planted, God may not have the power to change the oak tree once it's started to grow or the power to eliminate a parasite that threatens the tree's health.

What to Pray For

The deistic view of God and His creation may help you feel less singled out for cancer. It may help you to see that it has nothing to do with you personally. It may help you feel less abandoned by God; instead, it could help you feel that God is with you and suffers with you. But where does prayer fit in? What does it make sense to pray for? If you meditate, what can you hope to receive from God or the universe as you quiet your mind? Let's turn to these questions.

Most religious traditions teach that God is immanent in His creation and thus immanent in us. The Latin root of this concept of immanence is that God "dwells within" His creation. Many traditions resist the pantheistic notion that the universe *is* God. Instead, they speak of the "spirit of God" that dwells within His creation. The Protestant theologian Paul Tillich, for example, taught that the spirit of God empowers all of creation and keeps it going in a certain direction, thereby maximizing the potential for goodness.

It's a profound and powerful concept, I think, that the spirit of God dwells within us and empowers us to make good things happen. We have all done good works, and it may help to appreciate the underlying spirituality at work—that is, that we were *drawing upon* the spirit of God. Whenever we make something good happen—in our inner life, in our relationships, for the good of others, or for the planet—we are actually participating in God's plan, in His hope for creation. We can feel close to God in that sense.

What follows from this is a certain perspective on prayer, on what prayer is and what it means to pray or meditate. This point is supported by Christianity, Judaism, and deism, and it can also be found in Eastern religions and mysticism. Through prayer, we beckon something inside of us to come forth. Most generally, this "something" is the spirit of God, and most generally, it is there to bring goodness into our lives. But let's be more specific and relate it to the suffering cancer causes. I want to suggest five things to pray for.

Remembrance of All Good Things

When we are suffering, our world shrinks and we become preoccupied with our physical state. It can be an enormous challenge, in these moments, to remember all the good things that we have experienced in life. Pray for this memory; call it forth if you can. It can be of immense help to you. This memory is there and is one aspect of God's spirit within you. It's a resource that can offset the negative pull of your suffering. If you feel exhausted and depleted at the end of a long day, it can be difficult to remember even the good things that happened that day, such as a hot shower, the birds chirping outside, the comfort of a warm blanket . . . little things that can bring a smile to your face. Here again, you might want to pray for this memory to be there for you at the end of each day.

Gratitude

Remembrance of all good things can fill your heart with gratitude. One of my patients felt very grateful for her forty-four years of life until she was told that she had about three months to live. "My gratitude just evaporated on the spot," she said. That seemed totally understandable and valid. But then she prayed for gratitude, to be able to reclaim it and hold it close. And a remarkable thing happened. As soon as she uttered this prayer, she felt her gratitude return. It seemed the prayer was answered in the very act of the prayer itself. This helped her tremendously. She said it nudged her fear aside, made her feel less sorry for herself, and helped her to feel less depressed about dying young. "I feel more grateful than cheated," she said.

Courage

Courage enables us to face our fears instead of sticking our head in the sand. It can enable you to look squarely into the heart of your cancer, to metaphorically stare it down, and to respond with a tenacity of spirit *in spite of* your fear. It is not uncommon for people with cancer to be intimidated by it. They avoid thinking about it and avoid taking it on as a challenge. With courage, they can turn that process around. But oftentimes courage is not automatically given; we have to call it forth, to pray for it. One patient said he felt "terrorized" by his advancing melanoma. He wanted it to be over; "It will be a relief to die," he said. But when he prayed for courage, behold, there it was. He was amazed. He courageously pursued a new clinical trial where the chances of success were only 10 percent. He was aware of these odds and was able to face them. They did not intimidate him. They motivated him to respond aggressively and with hope that he could be among the 10 percent who survived.

Perspective

It is so easy to lose perspective when you are gripped with pain, nausea, fatigue—or when all the losses wrought by cancer just keep piling up. Perspective can be pushed aside by the sheer force of your suffering. One patient read that life expectancy in the 1800s was only in the mid-thirties, mainly because of the high mortality rate during childhood. Keeping this in mind made him more grateful for his fifty years. "It's all about perspective," he said. This kind of perspective has probably helped you as well. But it's easy to forget, and prayer and meditation can help to pull it back, back into the center of your mind, where it can help you to count your blessings and weather the storms of cancer. Everyone seems to know that perspective is important, but too often it is taken for granted or slips to the back of one's mind; it then loses its phenomenal power to bring comfort. It's definitely worth praying for.

Love

We have all read that God is love. I prefer to think that love is one aspect of God's spirit that dwells in all things. It may be that aspect that binds things together and creates order and beauty where chaos and randomness would otherwise prevail. Without love, perhaps there would be no hope for God's cause in creation. In human experience, we can be close to each other because of love, and through love we can transcend our self-centeredness. In the midst of suffering, it can be next to impossible to feel full of love, and for our love to flow out toward others and to all beings everywhere who suffer (as Buddhism teaches). Here too, this is something worth praying for. It may be a simple prayer, but then notice how it gets you out of yourself, out of your preoccupation with your own plight. I once led a support group of people in their thirties or forties who had less than a year to live. One member wanted to share something she had read, something that had helped her come to terms with her prognosis. "To love and be loved," she said, "that's the most important thing." That's what enabled her to feel fulfilled in her short life.

My Conclusion

From my background in philosophy and religious studies, and from my years as a psychologist working with people with cancer, I have my own beliefs about the point of this essay. I want to share those. Whatever is essential to you, in coping with your illness, you already possess. It is there in your heart, in the recesses of your mind, or in your soul. In your own way, you can beckon these to come forth. I have mentioned memory, gratitude, courage, perspective, and love; your own list could be shorter or longer, but it would be *your* list, your sense of what you need, something that you alone know. Whatever this essential truth happens to be, it can easily slip away, especially when all you want is relief from pain. I do not believe God can take away your pain. But He implanted in you all the resources you need to soothe your mental anguish and to find some sense of peace. These resources are in each of us. We are all children of God in that sense. Bad things like cancer can happen in God's creation. But when they do, God's spirit is there to comfort us and empower us to celebrate our existence in spite of our suffering. This is how God's spirit triumphs over the horror of cancer. This is how God's hope for us is not negated or defeated by cancer.

In 1945, a large clay jar was discovered in Egypt containing many writings from the Christian communities in the first and second centuries. One of these texts, called the Gospel of Thomas, quotes Jesus in saying number 70: "If you bring forth what is inside of you, it will save you." What is this thing inside of us, and how can it save us? Perhaps it speaks to the essence of who we are and how this essence can sustain us in our suffering. This suffering need not define the entire state of our being. You can be a grateful and loving being who is also suffering. You can still love life even while hating the conditions of your life right now. You can be saved by bringing forth resources and truths that are distinctly yours. These are God's gifts. We each have our own set. The God within can rescue you now and through all the trials that may lie ahead. A woman with brain cancer told me: "I feel I am in God's hands." She found a deep and sustaining peace in that.

EIGHT

On Coming to Terms with the Possibility of Death

CANCER IS CERTAINLY NOT ALWAYS a death sentence, and most people find it helpful to hold onto hope. But I have found that many cancer patients, especially those with a poor prognosis, think about their eventual death and whether they will be at peace with it when the time comes. They want to come to terms with it, as best they can, before they find themselves with only days or weeks to live. In this essay, I will discuss how patients I know have come to feel some sense of acceptance about their death, even though it may be several months away. Although it was a gut-wrenching process, it was not an impossible one. If you are struggling with this issue—wanting somehow to feel reconciled to dying, when the time comes, but not knowing how to get there—it may help to learn how other people with cancer have done it. If you have determined there is just no way, because dying feels so inherently unacceptable, it still may help to see how others have traversed this difficult path.

The phrase "coming to terms with death" means different things to different people, and often other phrases are used that convey the same general idea. These include "a sense of acceptance," "feeling reconciled," "being at peace with," "a feeling of equanimity about," "feeling okay about," "being resigned to," "giving in to," and "letting go." As you can see, there are different nuances of meaning in each concept, and I cannot think of a single conceptualization that captures all of them. Perhaps it's best to say that patients who have come to terms with their death do not feel they must continue to fight or protest it. It can be a long, heart-wrenching struggle to reach that point.

Another aspect of coming to terms with death is becoming less frightened or horrified by it. It would be difficult to approach death with a sense of peace or acceptance if you dreaded the process of dying. It may help to know that in the large majority of cases, the pain and suffering involved in dying of cancer can be effectively managed and controlled by the judicious use of opioids and other strategies. When the time comes, whether from cancer or some other cause, a hospice team or other palliative care specialists can play an invaluable role in helping with a peaceful death. Don't be hesitant to turn to them.

This essay is based not only on what patients in therapy have voiced to me, but also on interviews I conducted as part of a study with patients who were under fifty years old and had a poor prognosis. They sought to come to terms with their death as their cancer progressed and found that *perspective,* more than anything else, helped them in this process.

Six Perspectives

When I was at the UCSF Comprehensive Cancer Center, I knew many young patients who had a poor prognosis and who had managed over time to come to terms with the fact that they were likely to die within a year or two. I wanted a better understanding of how they had reached this point, an understanding that would help our team (and others in the field) to support these patients in the ways they needed. In a semistructured interview, twenty-five of these patients were asked to explain the kind of thoughts, emotions, beliefs, and experiences that had helped them in this process. The interviews were recorded and the transcripts were analyzed to identify common themes or factors (that is, certain thoughts, beliefs, or experiences) that helped these patients in facing an early death. Our research team identified six factors that were relevant to at least 50 percent of the patients interviewed. These were not the patients' *initial* feelings when first learning of their prognosis; these feelings evolved over time as they sought to come to terms with this prognosis.

1. Gratitude

This first factor was an astounding finding, attesting to the power of gratitude. It was discussed by 84 percent of the patients. They had looked back over the course of their lives and felt grateful for the number of years they had lived and for the positive experiences they had enjoyed. For most, feeling grateful helped to offset feelings of being cheated of additional life. It is common for older patients (in their seventies or eighties) to be grateful for a long life and for this to balance the negative feelings that death evokes. I learned from the interviews, however, that younger patients can feel grateful too, and to the extent they do, they feel less cheated. This was *the* most common factor mentioned by the patients I interviewed.

If you are a young person and have a poor prognosis, then you can look to the future and feel cheated of the life you will miss. But you can also look back at the life you have already had and feel grateful for that. Both perspectives are completely justified. One of the patients said that it was her choice—to look forward or to look back—and that she was choosing, and doing her best, to look back and take stock of what she could feel grateful for. Her gratitude provided comfort and helped ease the sting of an early death. She was only forty-two years old.

People who feel entitled to a good life, perhaps taking it for granted, seldom emphasize a sense of gratitude. Gratitude comes from seeing your good fortune in a world where no one's good fortune is guaranteed.

2. A Sense of Pride

This factor—a sense of pride in one's accomplishments or in the inner qualities the person had developed over the years— was mentioned by 80 percent of the patients. To feel proud of oneself is a positive feeling that can come from asking: "What have I done with my life? What have I made of myself?" The patients were not boastful about this; in fact, many were reluctant to use the word *proud*. They were more inclined just to say they felt good about certain things—usually something they had accomplished in work or in their personal lives, such as a long marriage, or being a good parent. When asked, however, they would say yes, it was a nice feeling of pride.

The idea of "a life" unifies our number of years into a whole. This construct has given birth to the question, What have we done with this thing called *our life*? Have we just lived, day in and day out, without any sense of unifying purpose that spans the years? But if we feel instead that we have put our lives to a positive purpose, then we can approach death with a deserved sense of pride. As with gratitude, this feeling can help soothe the emotional pain of dying young.

3. Religious Faith or Spirituality

Seventy-two percent of the patients said their religious faith or spirituality helped them come to terms with their prognosis. For many, it was the belief in some sort of afterlife, such as heaven or reincarnation. Some mentioned their spirit, essence, or soul—an aspect of their inner being that would live on in some spiritual form. Some had a basic belief in God's will or plan—a plan in which something positive would come from their death or how they dealt with it—and sought to accept their illness in that context. One patient mentioned the idea of *surrender* to God's will—of letting go and accepting whatever might happen.

Some patients said Buddhist beliefs and principles were helpful to them when thinking about death. In essence, these are beliefs about letting go because of the transitory nature of all that is. The following analogy conveys this essential teaching. Think of the ocean with countless individual waves and ripples on its surface. Underneath, there is only a vast ocean, a whole with no distinct parts. The distinct parts are on the surface only. These waves and ripples come into existence from the ocean, but are not the same as the ocean. They linger awhile on the surface and eventually go back into the deeper sea, the deeper whole wherein everything is one. All of nature, including ourselves, participates in this grand process of coming into being for a short while and then resolving back to our source. This conceptualization helped many patients feel it was okay and safe to let go.

I think the common denominator for all the patients who mentioned this factor was an appreciation that their individual lives were part of a larger reality or purpose (God's plan, the ebb and flow of the natural world, the oneness of being) and that feeling connected to this larger reality or purpose helped them to feel more accepting of their eventual death. "I am in

God's hands," one patient said. Some spoke of being held and protected, and that God would not allow them to suffer beyond their capacity.

4. Making Positive Changes

Sixty-eight percent saw their illness as an opportunity or call to make positive changes in themselves or their relationships, changes that would help them feel more fulfilled or at peace when death came. It has been said that it's not death per se that we fear, but rather dying when our lives are incomplete. This is why older people can more easily accept their deaths. The patients I interviewed were facing an early death, before their purposes had been met and before they felt personally fulfilled or complete. Still, they sought some sense of fulfillment, and took stock of how they might do that before it was too late.

These patients, as you may have noticed, were good at stepping back and taking stock of things. Perhaps this was *the* key to their ability to find some solace in facing death. Besides taking stock of things to be grateful for or proud of, they also did some serious soul searching. Some had to admit their life priorities had been askew. A common example was spending too much time at work and not enough time with family and friends. One person noted that he had lofty ideals: "I can talk the talk," he said, "but I don't really walk the walk." One patient said, "I need to be more true to myself, to what I really feel about things." Others mentioned making positive changes in their health habits to have the best quality of life for as long as possible. Some felt that they needed to deepen their faith and be closer to God; others mentioned that they wanted to figure out what they really believed. The most common feeling voiced by these patients was that their illness was a kind of wake-up call, an impetus to focus on what mattered most to them and to make changes that were overdue.

5. A Person's Legacy

This factor, discussed by 60 percent of the patients, concerned the importance of their legacy. As their illness progressed, they began to consider how they would be remembered, especially in terms of the positive contribution they had made to the lives of others, a contribution that would live on after they died. One woman, for example, talked about her artistic talent and love of doing watercolor paintings of mountain scenery. This was a cherished part of herself. It meant the world to her that her daughter was showing the same talent and interest. "That part of me will live on in her," she said. Another patient had held a managerial position in a large company and had gone out of his way, for many years, to play a positive role as a mentor for others on his staff. He sought to recognize and foster the special talent in each individual. After his diagnosis, several colleagues contacted him (some from as long as fifteen years ago) about the difference he had made in their professional lives. He choked up in telling me how much that meant to him.

It may seem grandiose for people to think about their legacy, or it may seem like a search for immortality. The patients I interviewed, however, seemed to have different motives. I think they were searching for meaning and found that in the positive difference they made in the lives of others. This was almost universally true of patients who had children. It makes sense, of course, when you are thinking about the end of your life, to think also about your life's meaning and purpose. Part of that meaning, as in Factor 2 just described, can be found in what you have accomplished. But it can also be found in ways you have enriched the lives of others because of what you have given of yourself.

6. Loving and Being Loved

The importance of loving and being loved was discussed by 52 percent. More than anything else, this (essentially) was what their lives were about. This is what connected them to family and friends, year in and year out. This was the most powerful and enduring source of meaning. Just to look back and know they had loved others, and others loved them, made it easier to face the prospect of death. "There's been a richness in my life because of that," one person said. Of course, they also felt grateful for this aspect of their life experience, which harkens back to Factor 1.

After doing these interviews, I explained the six factors in a support group of patients with metastatic melanoma. They all felt Factor 6 was the most important. "This is really what life is all about," one person said.

Why is that, do you think? Why does this particular assessment of one's life make the prospect of death less unbearable? One reason, I think, is that most people feel their worldly accomplishments have fallen short. They may compare themselves to others who were more successful. It can be consoling to see that certain worldly accomplishments really do not count for much; what is more important is the love in a person's life. The apostle Paul spoke of this in his famous passage in his first letter to the Corinthians. His point was simple and powerful: "If I have not love, then I amount to nothing." He felt this way despite all the other marvelous things he had accomplished.

Moreover, it speaks volumes about a person *to be loved by the right people and for the right reasons.* The right people are those in your life (not just anybody) whom you cherish. The right reasons are those aspects of your personality you hold dear, that define who you are. There are people in your life who know you in that way and love you because of these essential traits. As you read this, who comes to mind? Think about the many ways you have loved them, and how they have loved you. See whether that warms your heart and helps you feel more fulfilled or complete in your life.

My point in discussing these factors is not that you *should* feel the same as the patients I interviewed. No one should be so presumptuous as to suggest how another person should feel about his or her death. It is far too profound, too personal and private, and too complicated for anyone to burden you with a normative approach. Moreover, these six factors may or may not help with acceptance. At the very least, however, they might help balance the negative emotions that come naturally and appropriately when a person is forced to confront his or her death. Perspective is a powerful tool when needing to come to terms with things—perspective, that is, about your life journey and its meaning. A sense of fulfillment need not hinge primarily on how long you live. For many people, this sense is grounded in what they have done with the time they were given. If you can feel good about yourself and about your life, then you can feel (at least) less bad about dying and (at most) permeated with an abiding sense of peace.

Three Philosophical Concepts

There are three other ideas about death I want to mention. These have been voiced by patients of various ages I have known over the years. The patients who talked with me about this issue were being philosophical about it. That is, they were trying to articulate a basis or rationale for accepting death, one that makes sense but also feels right. These ideas may resonate with your own perspective on death or prompt you to feel more accepting about it.

I don't recall a patient ever saying to me, in private or in a support group meeting, "Here is the basis upon which I can accept my death." Instead, I have extrapolated the underlying rationale from what they said. Here is what I have gleaned from these discussions.

1. Death Is Inevitable

Some people try to accept death because it is inevitable. Their reasoning is straightforward and practical. Because they have to die someday, it is better to be at peace with it than depressed over it. This is a key in stoic philosophy—that is, that certain inevitable realities are bad enough already, and we should not make them worse by being depressed over them. (I elaborate on the stoic attitude or approach to cancer in "Giving Attitude to Cancer.")

2. Death Is Necessary

Some people have sought to be very philosophical about death in general, seeing it as a necessary part of the natural order of things. What would happen, for example, if living creatures were immortal, if there were birth but no death? One patient said he could not fathom living forever. The necessity of death, as part of the natural order, made it easier for him to accept his individual death.

As an aside, it may be helpful to consider the necessity of death in the evolutionary process. We are the product of evolution; countless living beings over millions of years have had to die in order for us to be here. This perspective can help us accept that our turn in this cycle will someday come.

3. Death Is Part of Life

I have heard this expressed many times. It is related to the idea that death is inevitable and necessary, but emphasizes *a life process* that involves birth, having a life, and then death. It's a perspective that says, simply: having a life means we have to die someday. It's part of the package. If we accept life on its own terms, then we should also accept death. The philosophical point is that we should embrace the whole process, not just the stage of being alive. Some people find comfort in being part of the natural order of things and thus sharing in the fate of all living beings.

Related to the idea that death is part of the package is the notion that death is the price that must be paid for getting to live or that it is part of the deal. In other words, we get something good (a life) but eventually have to pay for it by dying. This formulation only works, however, if one's life has been good. It's interesting to ask ourselves whether it is a worthwhile deal—that is, do the positive aspects of having a life *compensate* for having to die someday? If we can say yes to that, it means we have taken stock of these positive aspects and hold them close to our hearts as death approaches.

Many rationales for accepting death are intellectual and may or may not help with the emotional anguish of having to die. This is sometimes called the monkey on our back that we cannot shake. It is why Henry David Thoreau said most men lead lives of quiet desperation. It is why Freud said we must live in denial of our death because the emotions it evokes are so overwhelming. Our human consciousness is a gift of profound and sublime dimensions, but it also has a dark side: our awareness of our eventual death. What are we to do about this?

Religion, philosophy, and psychology can help, because our feelings about death depend on how we think about it. Our emotions do not arise in a vacuum. They arise on the basis of thought. We have thoughts about death, about what death is, and about the context in which we encounter it. The points we have discussed are essentially ideas—ideas about death that can help us come to terms with it. I think we each have a philosophy about death, or perhaps a theology about it. Perhaps this discussion has helped you to think about yours.

In the end, it can be good to face the prospect of death and to work on coming to terms with it, if possible. Too often, however, the kind of support that people with cancer receive goes in the opposite direction. Are people telling you, for example, to keep a positive attitude and a fighting spirit? Do they consistently focus on something encouraging or something that gives hope? Although all of this supports your optimism, don't you also need support in being realistic? It does not help when people counter your realism with an optimism that you feel, in all honesty, is unwarranted by your situation. Over the years, I have come to know thousands of people dealing with cancer; without exception, they all thought it *could* prove fatal. Most of them did not dwell on this, but the thought was there, always there in the back of their minds. What do you do with that thought? People will tell you to push it away, that it's negative and dangerous to think it. I don't believe this to be true. It's courageous to face it, and facing it is the first step toward coming to terms with it. It can also be the first step in taking nothing for granted and cherishing each day. Eventually, we are all confronted with the challenge of finding some sense of peace. Your loved ones may not realize you need more support in this process. If necessary, just tell them. It could pay off for you, and for them as well.

NINE

Cancer as a Gift?

MY FIRST REACTION TO the notion that cancer is a gift was one of disdain and contempt. This notion seemed to trivialize the suffering that cancer causes, and it seemed to place one more burden on patients who were trying to deal with their illness in all the right ways. Now, in addition to everything else, they were supposed to see their illness as a gift? I hated the idea.

Many people with cancer, however, have taught me that I was wrong. For them, there *was* something about having cancer that made it a kind of gift. To be more precise, they did not feel that cancer was a gift; rather, they felt there were certain aspects to having cancer that were actually good, and that those aspects could be called a gift. These positive aspects would not have occurred, they felt, had it not been for their cancer. Let me tell you what I have learned from others, and you can consider whether it applies to you.

More Appreciation

Normally we take so much for granted: our health, our loved ones, being loved, just being alive. A cancer diagnosis can be a kind of wake-up call to appreciate these things more fully, never again to take them for granted. Having cancer can be a gift in that sense.

A sixty-one-year-old man with pancreatic cancer told me, "You know, it's a shame it took cancer to hit me upside the head and show me how lucky I've been all my life." He said this new appreciation was not just a passing thing. It stayed with him day in and day out. Ironically, he said he was happier.

His new appreciation did not cancel out his dread about dying of cancer. It existed alongside his fear and sadness. It was genuine and real. He knew his prognosis was poor, and he was responding by taking stock of his life as a whole and feeling grateful. Even if he were cured, he said, he would not go back to taking things for granted. He said he would hang on to this gift for the rest of his days.

One woman told me she was looking out her kitchen window when her teenage son drove into the driveway, coming home from school. She had seen this many times, but all of a sudden it struck her—the total wonderfulness of having a son, a son who was getting an education that would carry him through life, a son who was home safe, a son who came home after school, a son whom she loved beyond all limits. He came in the kitchen and saw tears in her eyes. He asked what was wrong. She said: "You know, sometimes you cry because things are so right."

Living in the Present Moment

Our mind has a mind of its own, doesn't it? If left to its own devices, it will think about the past and the future, or about things that are going on currently in our lives, but rarely does it focus solely on the present moment. Just watch your mind and see what it thinks about. It will go all over the place. People who practice meditation try to quiet the mind and stay focused on the here and now. They just pay attention to what their body is experiencing in the moment. It breathes on its own.

It feels its weight on the floor or chair. It feels the temperature in the room. Just try to pay attention to all this and keep other thoughts away. It's hard to do. That's why people who practice meditation call it practice.

All we really have in life is our experience in the present moment. That is where we do all of our thinking. That's where things happen to us. All of our actions are there. We live in the present, but it goes by in an instant, doesn't it? No sooner do we think about the present than it's already in the past.

For many people, not being mindful of what they are experiencing in the present is not a problem. It can be nice to look forward to something in the future, or to remember something good that happened in the past. It can be fun to plan things, or to reminisce.

When a person has cancer, however, he or she can become more mindful of living in the present moment and regard that as a gift. Perhaps this is true for you. Like many people with cancer, your heightened awareness of your mortality—of cancer bringing an end to your allotted time—can make each additional moment more precious. You want to capture as much as you can from the here and now. You don't want it to slip away without your notice. You want to make the best of all the time you have. You don't want to waste it by worrying about things that you cannot control. Many people have told me these things.

A woman with cervical cancer was walking down the sidewalk on her way to our appointment. As she was walking, she said to herself something like this:

Here I am walking. My body knows how to do this. It's an amazing feat of balance and coordination. I have no idea how my body can do it. But who cares? Right now I feel the ground under my feet, a slight breeze on my face, warmth on my back from the sun. My belt feels a little too tight. I can see all around and hear many different sounds. There, a car just went by. It needed a new muffler. That is so cool: I heard the sound and knew it was too loud. Wait, now I am noticing that one shoelace is loose. Here I am stopping, and I can raise the foot with the loose lace, balancing on the other foot. What an amazing feat. My yoga class is paying off. And now my fingers seem to know how to retie the knot. They are doing it on their own. Another amazing trick. (I have no idea of how muscle memory works.) Wait, my mind is drifting to that question. Let's get back to walking, to being aware of what I am experiencing.

She told me this because she found it wonderful. She was taking a workshop in mindfulness meditation, trying to be mindful of the present as much as possible. She said she had walked down sidewalks all of her adult life and never before really captured the wonder of it.

There is a mindfulness meditation exercise wherein the instructor gives each person a raisin to eat as slowly as possible, being mindful of everything they are experiencing about the raisin. They close their eyes and take a full minute or more to eat one raisin. It's a real awakening for most people. They say they have eaten raisins all their lives, but never in this way, never being fully mindful of the taste, texture, and feel of it.

If your cancer has *not* made you more mindful and appreciative of the present moment, let's consider why. Perhaps you don't really "get it": the fact that you could die of cancer. Even if your prognosis is favorable, there is still some small chance that it could be fatal. Although the threat is small, the thing that is threatened (your life) is huge. When a person is *not* in denial about that, then I think they are brought around to a new appreciation of the time they have. When you know you may lose your life, then being alive right now takes on a new meaning and value.

I want to acknowledge, however, that there may be little to cherish in your present experience if you are feeling rotten, perhaps in a downward slide. You still may be able to find some moments to cherish. Even people in hospice care say that. Try to embrace whatever moments you can, moments of small comfort or special meaning. They can help to balance your suffering.

Realizing How Much You Are Loved

This is my hunch: people love you, but often they do not say those words, show their love, or say how much you mean to them. Cancer can change all that. Those who love you, when they are confronted with the prospect of losing you, often realize more acutely how important you are to them, and they want you to know that. When they see how you are suffering, they find themselves feeling a tenderness and caring for you that they want to express or show. They may just tell you directly. Even if it feels a little awkward, it can be very touching. Or they may demonstrate their love by wanting to be with you more than before, or by offering to do certain things for you—making a meal, walking the dog, going along to a doctor's appointment, shopping with you for hats or wigs, that sort of thing. They may just check in to see how you are. They may remember that scans are coming up. They may offer to go with you. They may remember to ask about the results.

What's more, old friends that you had lost touch with—former colleagues, old classmates, and other people you never thought you'd hear from again—are all of a sudden contacting you. Perhaps you had no idea of how much you mattered to them, or the effect you'd had on their lives.

Realizing how much you are loved can be one of the gifts that comes with cancer. It can seem sad, in a way, that it took cancer to bring all this to the surface. But it is also understandable. People are only human. Sure, before your cancer they were more or less taking you for granted. But now they have a new perspective.

But what if this does not apply to you? Suppose you are reading this and feeling only sad because your experience is quite different. Maybe you are feeling that people do not love you as much as you thought. It may seem that your cancer has scared people away. That can definitely happen. If this is true for you—if you are feeling more neglected than loved—then perhaps you are more aware of how much these other people mean to you. You may want to tell them that your cancer has prompted you to take an inventory, as it were, of the people who matter to you. You can tell them how they fit into that picture. Perhaps they didn't know. You can ask for their support. There is no sin in that. Your asking may not produce results. If they pull away, it will certainly hurt. But at least you'll know you have been real, that you were honest with your feelings and needs. Think about whether it may be worth the risk.

I know a man who prepared the most magnificent gift for his partner, who was dying from ovarian cancer. He contacted as many of her friends, colleagues, and family members as he could and asked them if they would write a short note telling her something that they remembered, something about her that touched them. He was swamped with wonderful vignettes and remembrances. Lots of old photos were sent as well. He put all this together in a binder and gave it to her for her birthday. She lay in bed, paging through the book, reading and crying as she went. She refused to part with it. She kept it on her nightstand and sometimes even held it as she slept. This material object, consisting of paper and ink and old photos, seemed to embody the love that so many people felt for her. It was the most touching gift imaginable. It gave her a peaceful death. It's hard to beat that.

Your Best Self Comes Forth

Cancer can bring out the best in people. When others rally around you in a selfless and patient way, it may occur to you that your illness has brought out the best in them. But what about this: has your illness also brought out the best in you? Many people with cancer feel that way. Perhaps they don't want to acknowledge it or seem boastful. But when asked about it, they admit to being surprised with the positive behaviors or attitudes that have emerged. This could be true for you as well. I don't mean you would shout from the mountaintops, "Hey, look at me: being strong, being courageous, showing love and appreciation." Maybe no one else would even know about it. But you would know, and that's what counts.

Let me tell you about Nancy. She was only thirty-four years old when she was diagnosed with breast cancer. It was an aggressive tumor that had invaded lymph nodes under her arm. Because of its size and location, a mastectomy was an option, but a lumpectomy might have sufficed. She chose the mastectomy. She also underwent radiation therapy and chemotherapy. She was fair skinned, and the radiation burned her badly. She lost her hair—the blond hair that she prized, that grew long and wavy, that she pampered with expensive shampoos and conditioners. Medications for nausea were only somewhat effective. She vomited every week after chemotherapy. She was already thin, but during her treatment she became skinny and bony in a way she detested. She was repulsed when she looked in the mirror. Disfigured, bald, skinny, burned. Dark circles under her eyes. She learned not to look at herself when she got out of the shower.

Nancy told me she had lived a charmed life before she was diagnosed. She was brought up in a loving, well-to-do family. She went to an Ivy League college. She was happily married to her college sweetheart. She was doing well in her career with an upscale advertising firm, and her future there was promising. She loved their small cottage-type home in the suburbs. It had everything but the white picket fence. She and her husband were planning to start a family in another year or two. But then she said something that surprised me. She said she was a "spoiled brat." She had always gotten everything she wanted.

Although she saw herself as a spoiled brat, she had not acted like one in response to her illness. She did not think: *How dare such a bad thing happen to me?* She did not feel entitled to special care or consideration. She cried as much as she needed to, but she did not overdo it to elicit more attention. She did not whine or complain. She did not run from harsh medical treatments. The threat of her cancer was met with the counterforce of her will and determination. Although she was repulsed by the damage done to her body, she regarded it as the price she was willing to pay in order to live. All of this revealed a wondrous strength of character.

The positive qualities that Nancy showed in dealing with her illness were not part of her self-concept, but they were part of her self. They were submerged, hidden even from herself, but came to the surface when she needed them. She did not take credit for them. She regarded them as a gift. They came forth because of her illness and became part of her identity.

Step back and look at how you've reacted to your illness. What do you see there? What does it say about you? Has anything new about yourself been revealed? Like Nancy, you may also see positive attributes that have come to the fore. If this is true, and if you can own these attributes as part of yourself, then they will be there for you in the future if the need arises.

Deepening Your Faith or Spirituality

Many people have ill-defined religious beliefs. Their faith is just there in the background and not particularly relevant to their day-to-day lives. Often it's the faith of their parents, who sought to instill it in them as children. Some aspects sank in but have lain dormant. When diagnosed with cancer, however, this under-the-surface faith comes forth and proves to be a reservoir of meaning, perspective, comfort, and strength. Their faith or spirituality is deepened in this process, a deepening that (they feel) would not otherwise have occurred. They feel their cancer was a gift in that sense.

Having cancer can cause people to turn to their faith, or perhaps to return to it if they have drifted away. One reason involves the search for meaning that comes with cancer. As people struggle to come to terms with their illness, they are often brought to the threshold of their religious faith. On a more emotional level, suffering creates a longing for comfort, strength, and hope. These elements often can be found in one's faith. The well-known psalm expresses it: "Although I walk through the valley of darkness and death, I fear no evil because you are beside me. Your rod and your staff comfort me." Many people find great comfort in this belief—the belief that God is with them or that they are in God's hands. It is the comfort of being held, protected, and sustained by a being of sublime love.

There is only so much we can do to alleviate our suffering; after that, we just have to live through it. This can require a fortitude of spirit, an inner strength that enables us to endure, to get back up when we feel like collapsing in a heap. For many people, this strength can be found in their faith. One person told me that he had not been to church for years. He was being treated for pancreatic cancer, and felt scared and weak—too weak to take on the challenge of fighting back. He went to church and just sat there quietly. Suddenly and mysteriously, he felt suffused with a sense of personal power to take on the difficult road ahead. "I don't know where that came from," he said. Moreover, the road ahead no longer seemed endless. As he was sitting there, he recalled the saying, "This too shall pass." It gave him hope. Everyone needs hope to forge ahead through all the ordeals that cancer can bring. Many people find this hope in their faith. Some believe that God will not allow them to suffer endlessly, or allow more suffering than they can handle. For others, their hope rests in their ultimate home, a home beyond this world, beyond their suffering.

The comfort, strength, and hope that people find in their faith are priceless gifts when dealing with cancer. Many people with cancer have discovered that. They find that their faith—inherited from their youth, neglected over the years, having receded into the background of their busy lives—is still there for them as a wellspring of the comfort, strength, and hope they so desperately need. By turning to this faith and delving into the rich wisdom that resides in their religious tradition, they feel a deepening of their faith and a new abundance of the grace it offers. Many have told me that this is one of the gifts that comes with cancer.

You may remember Gilda Radner from *Saturday Night Live.* She had ovarian cancer, which eventually took her life. According to her friend Joel Siegel, writing about his own cancer in *People* magazine in 2001, she joked about the various gifts that can come from cancer: "If it were not for the downside, cancer would be the best thing and everyone would want it." I love the humor in that, and also the wisdom. Because the downside to having cancer is so huge, no one wants it. But if you could somehow have cancer, without this downside, you might be happy for it because of all the ways it enriched your life.

TEN

My Interrupted Life: Jenny's Story

THIS IS THE STORY OF JENNY, a remarkable woman who was diagnosed with colon cancer at age forty-two. As you will see, she is remarkable in her ability to face harsh realities head-on, and to articulate the conflicts and dilemmas that bounced around in her mind. Her story, I believe, speaks to the experience of many people with cancer.

In reading her story, you'll see how Jenny dealt with many of the themes discussed in this book—anxiety, existential dilemmas, gratitude, family communication, and more. She dealt with everything in her unique way, just as everyone with cancer has his or her own way of dealing with all the trials that face them personally. Perhaps Jenny's story will resonate with yours, reminding you that you're not alone in your journey—a realization that can also be found in support groups. Perhaps the way she communicated with her husband, son, and friends about certain issues will give you ideas for how to communicate with your loved ones. Or perhaps Jenny's story or way of thinking is vastly different from yours, and you can learn something by comparing and contrasting your viewpoint with hers. Perhaps you'll take away this point: each journey is unique, and there is no wrong way to traverse it. This is Jenny's story. Maybe hers will inspire you to write down or share your own.

Jenny allowed me to tape-record some of our sessions, and she copied some of her journal entries for me to read. I also have notes from our therapy sessions and from the support group that she attended, and that I led. I borrowed from this material to piece together her story. The story is told in the first person, as if she were telling it to me, because much of it was that way. My questions or interjections, when relevant, are placed in parentheses. Often I use her exact words, but just as often I paraphrase or edit her words to capture the flow of her story. To protect her privacy, and that of her husband and son, I have altered information that might disclose her true identity.

It Began

It began on my toilet in our downstairs bathroom. I went to flush the toilet and jerked back with a start. There was blood there, lots of it. It must be hemorrhoids, I thought. But do they bleed like that? I guess they must. I paused before flushing, just staring at all that blood. Then it was gone.

My concern was not gone, however. I didn't tell my husband, Gary. Knowing him, he'd get all worked up over it. And my son Jared, the teenager, well of course I didn't tell him. "Too much information, Mom." That's what he'd say. When I had to go again, I was afraid to look in the bowl. I sat there, trying to get my nerve up. Finally I looked. Hah, not a drop of blood. You see, just hemorrhoids or some flukey thing.

Three days later, there it was again. Bright red blood. I've never heard of hemorrhoids doing that. I honestly can't remember if I was thinking it might be cancer. But I must have been—I mean, why else was I worried that first time? I knew I needed to get it checked.

I told my doctor about the bleeding. He asked if there was any colon or rectal cancer in my family. That really hit me. I mean, the first thing I thought was hemorrhoids. The first thing he says was cancer! I didn't think it was in the family. So he said it must be hemorrhoids. Hah, what a relief! He said I was too young for that kind of cancer. He prescribed some suppositories for hemorrhoids. That was it.

(*He didn't examine you?*)

No, I guess he didn't think it was necessary. It was fine with me.

There was still blood, about every other time. *My hemorrhoids must need a different kind of suppository*—that's what I thought. Or maybe it was cancer. I thought that too. Two weeks went by. Finally I had to tell Gary. I mean, I was keeping a big secret from him. But you know, it was hard being alone with this secret. I wanted him to know. He asked all about it— you know, how often there was blood, what the doctor said, was there any pain, that sort of thing. I told him I was floored when the doctor had asked about cancer. "Cancer!" he said. "Can cancer cause bleeding like that?" I just looked at him. "I think so." I said it in such a serious way. It surprised me. Gary could tell too. He asked why I hadn't told him earlier. I said it was probably nothing and that I didn't want him to worry. You know what he said to that? At first he was a little sarcastic and said "Oh, I see. All this time you have been worrying about cancer *and* worrying about how I'd feel." Then his voice softened and he looked me in the eye. He said, "Sweetheart, let's worry *together* about this cancer thing, if we have to. We'll tackle it together, if we have to, okay?" Those were almost his exact words. I started to cry.

We went back to my doctor, told him about the bleeding, and asked that he take a look. While he was examining me, he said that he couldn't see any hemorrhoids. Gary and I shot each other a look. We were thinking the same thing. He asked my doctor what might be causing the bleeding. My doctor said it could be a tear in the rectum that surgery could fix. He said he would order a colonoscopy for me. Damn that Gary, he had to ask if it could be cancer. My doctor said cancer was not likely. I was young and had no family history. He reiterated that point.

I don't know if I can tell you about the colonoscopy without crying. I was watching it on the monitor. At first my insides were all pink and healthy looking. But farther up the colon . . . (*her voice was choking now*) . . . there it was . . . (*pause*) . . . it looked so ugly and nasty, black and purple mostly, some mucous or pus on it, I don't know. It was about the size of a walnut I'd say. The picture of it is right here in my mind—emblazoned on my mind, I think that's the phrase. I started to have a panic attack, I guess, so they gave me more anesthesia and that's all I remember. They took a biopsy of it while I was out. I woke up in the recovery room. Gary was there, holding my hand. He had tears in his eyes. The doctor was there, telling him the news. "It looked like cancer. It was sent to pathology, and we should know in a few days."

Then Gary—damn him, bless him—asked, "If it's cancer, how bad did it look?" "It looked bad to me," I blurted out. The doctor said it all depended on whether it had grown through the wall. I'd have to have surgery to find out. This was the start of the never-ending, agonizing waiting. Wait for pathology, wait for surgery results, wait for scan results . . . wait and see if you will live or die.

Gary drove us home. We were quiet, both stunned I guess. Then he asked, "Did you really see it?" The dam burst and I just sobbed and sobbed. I've thought about it since, that question, the best possible question . . . the question that showed he knew what I was thinking, the image I kept seeing in my mind, that horrifying sight that he was not afraid to know about. A friend asked me later, "Didn't it upset you, to be reminded of that frightening sight?" I said no, I was already thinking it, seeing it right there. It looked so evil. He didn't remind me of *it*. He reminded me that I was not alone. He wished that he had seen it too. He said something like that. He didn't want me to be the only one living with that memory, with that image in my mind.

Gary was quiet the next day. "A penny for your thoughts," I said, like a little girl. He said he didn't want to tell me. He didn't want to sound pessimistic. "But the truth is," he said, "I'm thinking 'What if?' What if you die? I can't stand that thought." His voice cracked when he said that. I don't think I ever felt so loved. Isn't that odd? He's told me countless times that he loves me. But there he was, choked with emotion, because my death, if it came to that, would just rip him apart.

The next day the dreaded call came. It was colon cancer, and I was being sent to a GI surgeon. I asked if they could tell how serious it was, from what the pathologist saw. I was searching for something hopeful to hang onto, like maybe it was just a baby colon cancer that had not learned the nasty ways of grown-up tumors. My doctor said they'd remove the tumor along with a section of my colon. That would show if it was caught early. That's all he could tell me.

Gary and I got on the Internet to read about colon cancer. We found the Johns Hopkins website and thought we could trust that. I started to read about the stages of colon cancer. When I got to Stage 3 I broke into a cold sweat. It said that if the cancer got into lymph nodes you could die. It could spread to the liver or lungs. The chances were about 35 percent, on average. I was thinking, *What? Isn't there a chemo to cure it?* I laugh now, seeing how naïve I was. Well, it said there was chemo for it, but it was pretty clear it might not work. It wasn't that blunt, but I was getting the picture. When I got to Stage 4 I had to stop. I didn't want to go there. I was thinking, *I don't need to learn about that. It won't get that far.*

I felt mixed about it, like it could go either way. I was scared, but hopeful too. I mean if you asked me, "Do you think you'll die of colon cancer?" I'd have said no. Hmm, that's interesting... I just had a hit of anxiety in saying that. We talked about that in the support group, that it feels like you're asking for trouble if you go around saying you are going to beat it. I mean you might not, you could die, that'd teach you a lesson about being too bold or too confident. That's how you put it in our meeting, I think.

Anyway, I didn't read about Stage 4. It's probably when it gets into your brain or something, when you are really toast. I didn't know how much I wanted to know. Part of me thought, *Hey, come on now, face it. Don't be afraid of it. Don't be a sissy.* But then I'd think, *What's the point of living in fear? I am scared enough already. I need to have hope, be filled with hope, not filled with fear.*

(*Is it true that if you knew all the stages and all the statistics, that it would undermine your hope?*)

Well, that's what I didn't know. I didn't know how bad the statistics were. If they were really bad, then maybe I'd rather not know. That "ignorance is bliss" thing. But if they were really bad, maybe I should know to prepare myself. And I wondered about Gary. Would he want to know my prognosis? I thought so. He's that way. Get all the cards on the table. That's what he'd say. If it's bad, I can see it now, we'd both break down, be a puddle on the floor. Maybe that'd be okay, to cry it out together. Sounded like doom and gloom, though.

It Led to Limbo

The surgeon said I should have a CT scan before the surgery. He said it would show if the cancer had spread anywhere, like to my liver. That Gary, sometimes I want to muzzle him. He had to ask if I'd still have the surgery if the cancer had spread. He told me later that he was just thinking, *Why did I have to have the scan first?* It must be because the doctor needed a green light to proceed, implying—this is what Gary said, if you can believe it—implying that if it had spread, the surgery would not do any good because it was too late for that. Like I said, he wanted all the cards on the table. I wasn't sure I did, though. When he asked that question, my anxiety shot right up. Before I could say, "Uh, excuse me doctor, you don't have to answer that," the doctor replied they'd probably do chemo first, to get it under control, and then do the surgery later. Hah, I liked that answer, that "get it under control" part—it gave me a shot of hope, that this cancer could be treated.

He also wanted to check my CEA before surgery. (*CEA is a tumor marker in the blood for colon cancer.*) This time I asked the question—wanting to show that I was brave too, not just Gary—whether I'd still have the surgery if the CEA was high. He said I definitely would, and they'd expect the CEA to go down after the surgery, assuming that the tumor in my colon was the culprit, putting out the CEA in my blood.

• • • THREE WEEKS LATER • • •

I'm feeling pretty up today. The CT scan was all clear. But what a harrowing experience. They're looking for mets, pure and simple. They're looking for what they might find if they look carefully enough. I'm lying there hoping they don't look too close. Isn't that silly? You should want them to look closely so they don't miss anything. That seems logical, don't you think? But I gotta tell you: at least for me, logic was out the window. There was no way I was thinking logically about it. I wanted them to take a quick look and find nothing. Isn't that bizarre? And of course you don't know what they're seeing. You just lie there praying they find nothing, nothing but normal guts and stuff, no little tumors anywhere. Oh, I almost forgot the worst part. They were scanning an area on my belly and said they needed to go back and take some more pictures, to get a better look. I was thinking, *Holy shit, they see something!* I felt light-headed and sick to my stomach. Oh, and afterward, you try to get a clue from the technicians. They were so poker-faced about it. "How'd things look?" I asked them that. One of them said something like, we don't really know, we're not trained in that. The radiologist has to review the films. I'm sure he has said that a thousand times. And what kind of talk is that, any-way? "The radiologist will review the films." In other words, the radiologist will tell you if you'll live or die. Have a nice day. That's how it felt.

• • • ONE MONTH LATER • • •

It's ironic. It was so great to have the surgery behind me. I remember saying to the tumor, right before they put me out: *Goodbye damn cancer. Be gone Satan.* And when I woke up, I knew it was gone. It was such a great relief. I guess I was kid-ding myself.

My surgeon called a few days later with some bad news. Some really bad news. He didn't say it that way, but that's what it was. Well, maybe it's not so bad. I don't know what to think about it. The tumor had grown through the wall and they found a little bit of the cancer in some of the lymph nodes nearby. Three lymph nodes, they said. They removed twelve, but it was only in three. Did I say "a little bit of cancer"? That's cute. Sounds pretty harmless, putting it that way. What he said was "microscopic involvement." That's why it didn't show on the scans. But I know what it means. It means Stage 3. It means I am in limbo now. Frozen in limbo, that's how it feels. Having to wait . . . it could be years of waiting.

(*Why do you feel frozen?*)

Because it makes no sense to have future plans, or even to look forward to something, like Jared graduating and going to college—it could all come to naught, just like that. The cancer comes back and all bets are off. Everything goes out the window. I feel I have to put my life on hold now—that's it.

• • • THREE WEEKS LATER • • •

Yesterday we saw Dr. Nelson, the oncologist here, supposedly the colon cancer guru. He said I needed chemo just in case the cancer had spread. "Just in case"—that's how he put it. Gary—this was typical—asked if the chemo would work. I mean, if it did spread somewhere, would the chemo kill it off? I was like a deer in the headlights waiting for the answer to that. I could tell Dr. Nelson was uncomfortable in telling us. He said it might work, but it might not work. It could still come back, despite the chemo. You get the picture here? I have to poison my body with drugs that I might not even need, and even if I do need them they might not work.

I must be sounding pretty negative or cynical about all this, huh? I read somewhere that cancer patients should "embrace" their chemotherapy in a positive way. I mean, it *does* offer hope. It gives me that 65 percent chance I read about in Stage 3. Anyway, this idea of embracing the chemo, I'm trying to get with that. I mean, if I'm hugging the toilet and puking my guts out—damn, you see how negative I can be?—I guess it'd help to say, Hey, bring it on. It's strong medicine. It's making me sick and killing those cancer cells. I mean, what if it didn't faze me? I'd think they gave me the wrong chemo or too weak a dose.

• • • THREE WEEKS LATER • • •

Want to know what a weird thought I had, when I was in for chemo? There were lots of patients there, and when Dr. Nelson came out to get them, he'd be carrying their chart. And lots of those charts were really thick, like almost two inches. That really struck me. I was thinking, those people must have been dealing with cancer a long time, like for years maybe, in order for their file to be so damn thick. I mean, thick is good, right? My chart only had a few pages in it. Obviously I was a newcomer. But I was thinking, *See, not everyone dies of cancer right away, and maybe not at all. These people with thick files, I bet they're basically cured but just come in for checkups.* It gave me hope. I want a thick chart someday.

· · · THREE WEEKS LATER · · ·

My CEA is looking good. Before the surgery it was up to 8, which isn't too high in the scheme of things. That's what we read. It's back to normal now, which is really good. I mean, if the cancer was hiding out somewhere, the CEA would still be high. So there's a good chance they got it all. That's what my surgeon said. It had such a nice ring to it. "I think we got it all," that's how he worded it. I'll never forget that. I was so relieved, silly me. Since then I've learned what it really means. It means they got all the "gross tumor"—what a perfect phrase—they could see right there. What they don't say right then, so they don't scare the bejesus out of you, is that some of it might have gotten away, like into your bloodstream—and if that happened, well, let's not go there. They certainly don't get into that, at least not then.

The plan now is to check the CEA every three months or so. If it stays normal, I'm in good shape. If it starts going up . . . (*pause*) Well, if it stays normal, I can relax for at least another three months. I get to live three months at a time.

Dilemmas in Limbo

• • • FOUR MONTHS LATER • • •

You know Jerry in our support group? I couldn't believe all the *extra* things he's doing, like no more red meat, doing yoga, meditating every day, taking Chinese herbs. I didn't want to admit it then . . . but I'm not doing any of that stuff. Friends, people in my family, they all have advice about what I should be doing. Some new drug or vitamin or something. My sister heard somebody on the radio talking about a psychic healer in Brazil or somewhere. She called me right up and said I gotta go see this guy.

I'm not going for that. I'm not Jerry. I'm doing chemo—isn't that enough? I get through my chemo days, go to work, shop for groceries, help Jared with his homework if he lets me, do the laundry—you know, I'm trying to go on with my normal life. I'm not taking time out to visualize my natural killer cells attacking those weak, cowardly cancer cells hiding in some tissue cave here or there. That's what the chemo is for. But then I think, *If it comes back, will I blame myself for not doing more? Will I regret I didn't do more to fight it? Maybe it would have made a difference, if I had meditated or gone to yoga class, things like that. Maybe I wouldn't be at Stage 4, facing death and all. Maybe Jared wouldn't have to lose his mother.* But I'd never really know, right? I mean, all the things that Jerry is doing, maybe it doesn't really help. But I'd have that question gnawing away at me. I guess if you do those extra things, and if it comes back anyway, at least you wouldn't be blaming yourself or having that regret. I wonder if that is why Jerry is doing it.

• • • FIVE MONTHS LATER • • •

Gary and I were complaining the other evening that lots of our friends don't seem to get it: that my cancer could come back at any moment and I'd be in a heap of trouble. Since I've finished chemo, and my scans are all clear, they seem to think my cancer is behind me now and it's time to stop worrying about it. A few days ago I had a headache and said to my sister, half joking, that it could be a brain tumor. I don't mean that I thought that it *was* a brain tumor, only that it *might* be. Anyway, I told my sister and she really scolded me. She thought I was being way too negative. She said something like, "There's no sign of it anywhere. It's gone. You can stop worrying about it. You should celebrate being healthy again." Words to that effect. When I'm positive, people are all for that and say, "You go girl! You are beating this thing!" But if I'm sad or worried, then there's an awkward silence . . . like they disapprove and don't know what to say. It makes me feel like I'm only supposed to be positive, in their view. It seems like they don't get it—that it's still hanging over me day after day. Gary gets it completely. He's not that way at all. But he's the exception.

That night in bed, after the lights were out, I had the most disturbing thought: *Maybe I don't get it either, the fact that I could die in a year or two? I mean, I say those words, but do I really get what that means? If I really got it, I think I'd be a basket case.* It points to that question we discussed in group once, about what it means to die. Intellectually, we know what it means. But when you really think about it, it seems too horrible to comprehend. Anyway, I was thinking I should lighten up on everyone else.

(*I'm struck by the fact that you want very much to get it. Why do you suppose that is?*)

Do you mean that I might be expecting the worst?

(*It could be that, but it might be you just want to be pre-pared, in case it comes to that.*)

You know, that's typical of me. I hate to be caught off guard. If I was all positive about things, and then my cancer came back, I'd feel like what an idiot! Why did I have my head in the sand? I'd rather face the dark side, if you know what I mean. If it comes back, I want to have a response all prepared and ready. I am rehearsing in my mind how I'd react.

(*That response you are rehearsing—can you tell me what that is?*)

Well, I guess I really can't predict it; I'd probably freak out no matter how prepared I was. But I'd like to be somewhat Buddhist about it . . . you know, accept it as part of life . . . the transitory nature of life. That's what I'd like, if it's possible. If I am going to die, I'd like it to be peaceful. I don't know how to get there, but that's what I'd like.

• • • FOUR MONTHS LATER • • •

That discussion in our group last week, what Carol said about crossing a bridge if and when you come to it, that really got me thinking. I'm always dreading that bridge, but may never come to it. What's the point of that, I wonder? Why not live as if I'm going to be an old woman wearing purple someday? Why not go on with my life in a happy way? If the cancer comes back, deal with it then. I sometimes wish I didn't know what I know.

(*Is there any advantage to knowing what you know?*)

Well, I'm all for being prepared. I guess there's a plus side to that; not being blindsided and all. I don't take things for granted like I used to. I guess that's a plus too. Jared had some friends over and they were playing ping-pong. I was watching him and just thinking, *I love this boy, and I love what he's doing right now, having fun, having friends.* He's good at ping-pong too. That was great to see. I would not have given these things a second thought before. My sister and her husband were over for dinner last week. When they were leaving, I hugged them goodbye and said, "I really love you two." Tears came to my eyes. I never said that before. My sister got tearful too and hugged me again. She said, "Try not to worry. You'll be okay."

Falling from Limbo

• • • FIVE MONTHS LATER • • •

I got some bad news, I think. My CEA went up to 9 since three months ago. When Dr. Nelson told me, I felt sick to my stomach. He told me not to jump to conclusions—something like that. He said lots of things can elevate the CEA, things other than colon cancer. He wants to check it again next month. If it goes up some more, he said we should do a CT scan. So I have to sweat it out for a month. But I gotta tell you, there was a look on his face . . . he didn't smile that same smile he usually has. He tried to put a positive spin on it. But I think he was worried and tried to hide that.

When I got home I told Gary. He just looked at me and said nothing for a few seconds. There was a look on his face. It spoke volumes, but I can't put the right words to it. A seriousness came over him . . . like when I told him what the cancer looked like. I sat on our sofa and he came over and sat on the coffee table, right in front of me. I was looking down, afraid to look at him. I did not want to see that look . . . the pain on his face, the pain I was causing him. I was so sorry for him and felt guilty too. I wanted to tell him it was probably a false alarm. I wanted to lie but I couldn't. He lifted my chin up and looked right at me. He was fighting back tears and biting his lip. Then he asked, "What do you think it means?" If I thought it meant cancer, then he'd follow my lead. He always wants to be where I am. Not ahead of me, but not dragging up the rear either. I said something like, "I think it means trouble, but maybe not. We have to wait a month for the next test." He said okay to that. There was a tear on my face, and he wiped it away with his thumb. Then he kissed his thumb and placed it on my lips. We both smiled at that. Sounds a little corny now, but it was sweet then.

• • • FIVE WEEKS LATER • • •

I think I'm in real trouble. The CEA went up to 11. This time Dr. Nelson did not hide his concern. I could tell right when he walked into the room. Gary was with me. Dr. Nelson said, "I'm sorry Jenny, but the CEA is up a little higher this time." Those words hit like a shock wave. I think I even backed up. Ha, that's funny in a way. It's like I wanted to put some distance between myself and the news. I asked if something else could cause that, for it to go up to 11. I was searching for hope. We both knew that. He said it was possible, but it could be a recurrence too. He said he wouldn't place a bet either way. I think it was a lie, but a good lie. We both knew it was a lie, I think. I like him. I know he cares about me. He didn't want to floor me with bad news. Gary clenched his jaw and hit his fist on his knee. Then he looked up and his eyes were just a puddle. He was blinking the tears away. It's funny I remember that so clearly.

When we got home we told Jared. He was playing a game on the computer. We said we needed to talk with him about something serious. He's a teenager, remember, and he didn't want to be interrupted. He was in the middle of a game and couldn't put it on pause. He said "In a minute, okay?" We said okay, that we'd be waiting in the family room. Then he glanced up and saw the look on our faces. "I'll stop now," he said. He's such a sweetheart in that way. He can sense our emotions a mile away. We told him what the CEA was, and that it was normal but then went up to 9 and then to 11, and that I needed to have a CT scan to see if the cancer was back. We just put it right out there in a matter-of-fact way. I think his eyes opened wider as he took in this news. Right away he asked the right question, the question that Gary and I had too. If the cancer was back, couldn't it be cut out, just like before? I glanced over at Gary. I guess I wanted him to answer that. He said it depended on where the cancer was, and the CT might show that. Jared seemed fine with that; he seemed to feel that we shouldn't jump to any conclusions until the scan results. But Gary wanted him to know something else, and I guess I did too. If it came back, Gary said, it means the chemo didn't kill it all, and it might be in other places too small to show up on the scan. You know Gary—he says it straight. I was wondering, *Does Jared need to know that now?* Well, it was too late, now he knew. Jared looked back and forth at both of us. "What are you saying?" he asked. Can you believe that? He's only sixteen. He wanted to cut to the chase. I mean, what *was* Gary saying? What did he want Jared to know? That I could die? If the chemo didn't work, does that mean there's no stopping it? I can't believe that. . . . Anyway, Gary said something like, "If the chemo didn't work, then Mom's in trouble." Jared was now staring at Gary with a laser look. He was perfectly still. Just that wide-eyed laser look, the one that means business. "What do you mean, that Mom's in trouble?" That's what he asked his dad. I saw these two men, the hub of my life, and felt like a new bond was growing between them, one that had to do with me, with something they shared—their fear of losing me, I think. That's how they are, those two. Gary said the chemo I took had the best chance of killing the cancer. If it was only in one spot, maybe surgery would work. Maybe other chemos would work. There were still lots of weapons to use. Then he said, and I remember these words: "But Jared, sweetheart, Mom could die, that's what I mean by trouble." He hasn't called Jared "sweetheart" since he was five, maybe six. Jared did not seem to object. But then he yelled at Gary, and he was crying too: "Mom's not going to die, Dad!" And he stormed out.

• • • TWO WEEKS LATER • • •

There are two small spots in the liver. New spots. Nothing else anywhere, which is good. Just those liver mets. I read the report. So did Gary. There was a bunch of radiologist jargon that I didn't understand, in the description of these spots. Nodules, that's what they were called. At the bottom were the words "suspicious for metastatic disease." That I understood. Pretty blunt. They say "suspicious" because they don't know for sure. But who are they kidding? I mean really? Both spots were about the size of a pea. Dr. Nelson said they'd be hard to biopsy. He wants me to try another chemo. Oh, he wants me to see a surgeon too. He said it might be operable. If nothing else showed up, maybe surgery would be the way to go. You know, they can remove a piece of your liver and it will grow back. Isn't that something? I asked if the new chemo could kill them off, those two mets, so I wouldn't need surgery. I could tell he didn't like that question. There's a chance, he said. But I could tell. He looked away. He wasn't too hopeful about that. But he didn't want to say that flat out.

Jared was still at school when we got home. I went to a website I'd seen before, where they discussed surgery for liver mets. It said sometimes colon cancer only spreads to the liver, and surgery might be possible depending on where it is. But then it said, get this, that you could be cured. It actually said "cured." There was a 10 to 15 percent chance. I mean we are talking about Stage 4, which I thought was incurable, plain and simple. I showed it to Gary, that part about a cure being possible, to make sure I was reading it right. You know, if you think it's going to get you, sooner or later, I mean if they don't find a better treatment, and you read a 10 to 15 percent chance of a cure, that's huge!

Anyway, we heard Jared drive into the garage, and I think we kind of braced ourselves, because we had to tell him. I mean we didn't *have* to, but I guess it's our policy now, to be up front with him. You won't believe this, but he comes in, says hi, and heads for his room. Then he does this U-turn and asks if I had any news about the scans yet. Isn't that amazing? I mean, it was on his mind, that my scan results were coming. He's tuned in, that kid, to the horrible drama we are all living through. I told Jared the whole thing. Well, not really. I didn't dwell on what Stage 4 means and all that. I tried to be more positive—you know, that it was only in the liver, very small, maybe surgery would do the trick, a cure was possible, all of that.

(*How did he react?*)

He didn't seem surprised about the liver mets. I mean we had pretty much told him that we expected some kind of recurrence, because of the CEA. What he was really feeling inside, I don't know. I think he's scared, but has hope too. Just like Gary and me. Gary and me, and our boy.

• • • ONE MONTH LATER • • •

I was in a funk yesterday and went to my journal to write it out, to get to the bottom of it. I sat there with my fingers on the keyboard, waiting to see what came. I was expecting some doom and gloom to spew out, but instead, my fingers told me to celebrate life. It's not an original idea, of course. I mean, we have all heard that many times, that we should celebrate life. This time, though, on this occasion, this phrase spoke to me personally. It wasn't just a nice idea. It seemed to be the answer to the funk I was in. Right away all kinds of memories came flooding in . . . all kinds of reasons for celebrating life. I thought of the night Gary proposed to me. It was exhilarating. I thought of the morning we watched to see if the test tube turned blue, you know, that home test to see if you're pregnant. We had been trying forever to get me pregnant. We were crying and laughing, both of us. Then we hugged for the longest time. I remembered that scene, a clear picture of it. I remembered a Christmas morning when I was young. My sister got roller skates. I really wanted those. My mom saw me looking at those skates. I can remember this like it was yesterday. She said, "Jenny, we got roller skates for you too." She explained that the store didn't have my size, so they were ordered, and weren't in yet. What's funny is, I never knew if that was true. I got my own skates a few days later. I always smile when I remember that—thinking that my mom might have made it all up on the fly, seeing that I was envious of those skates. All these memories came pouring in . . . memories of things to celebrate and be grateful for.

The Dangle of Hope

• • • FOUR MONTHS LATER • • •

[*In our support group meeting, Jenny told the group that her scans showed a small increase in the size of the liver nodules but there was no sign of metastases anywhere else. Moreover, the surgeon said the liver metastases were in an area that could be removed and would regenerate. Surgery was scheduled in three weeks.*]

It's a funny thing, having hope but telling myself not to have too much hope. Then I think, *Screw it! I am full of hope and that's that.* You know I like to be prepared for bad news. Okay, I'm prepared. I mean I've been living with death staring me in the face for several months now. I've tried to get ready for the end, tried to get my mind in a peaceful place. But screw that too! I'm sorry, but I have real hope this time. This surgery could cure me. It's scary to say that. It's like setting myself up. I tell myself: *Lay low. Don't go around all pumped up with hope, only to have cancer come back to put me in my place.* It's better to lay low, I said. But screw that too! I'm sorry, but we're talking about a possible cure here. It's only in one part of my liver, and surgery will get it all. That's my new mantra. It may be false hope, I know. But right now I am going for it. Gary, however, is not on the same page this time. You know what he said? He said he couldn't stand to get his hopes up, and then have to relive the horror of losing me, if the cancer comes back. "I can't go through that again." Yes, he's hopeful too, but in a guarded way.

(*What about Jared?*)

Oh, he's acting like it's a done deal, that I'll be fine. That's his position, until he learns otherwise. That's what he said.

• • • TWO MONTHS LATER • • •

[*Jenny's surgery went well and she took a month off to recover. She emailed the group that she was doing fine and thanked them for their concern and support. She came back to the group last week, which was the first time I saw here since the surgery. Her CEA was back in the normal range. The following week, we had a private session to check in.*]

It's back to limbo, right? The group thought so too. (*sighing*) More waiting now to see if it shows up anywhere else. Jonathan thought that if it had spread elsewhere it would have shown up by now. I liked that point. Maybe it's more hopeful than I think.

(*You said in our meeting that you were guardedly optimistic. Is that right?*)

Yeah, guardedly optimistic, that's right, that's where I am. But to tell the truth, I felt guilty saying that, guilty about the whole thing, about maybe being cured now. Ally was sitting across the room from me. Sitting there with mets to her lung. How was she supposed to feel? She might have been thinking, *Well, goodie for you. You might be cured. What about me?* I mean, I don't think she was thinking that. But *I* was thinking that. I wanted to hold back in talking about being hopeful or whatever. I didn't want to sound presumptuous. I think that's why I made a big point about being in limbo again.

(*Do you feel less in limbo than you said? I mean, maybe you really feel you have one foot out the door, leaving limbo behind?*)

That's such a hard question. I mean, how do I *really* feel? There's how I feel—which is full of hope, even excited about having my life back—and then there's how I *should* feel—which is much more guarded. Much less presumptuous.

$$\bullet\ \bullet\ \bullet$$

I will end Jenny's story at this point. She stayed in our group for another two years. Her cancer never recurred during that time. She continued to be optimistic, but guardedly so. She continued to struggle with how she should feel.

I was reluctant to tell her story because it has a happy ending. You might be reading this and thinking, just as Jenny was worried about what Allison was thinking, *Well, goodie for her. She was lucky. How's that supposed to make me feel, since I am not so lucky?* If this is true, that your luck has not been so good, then no one would blame you for feeling bad when you hear a story like Jenny's. I don't see any easy way around that. Some people have good luck. They rejoice in that but also feel guilty because their good luck can make other people with cancer feel bad in comparison. Some people have bad luck. They have to deal with that as best they can. They hear stories about cancer survivors and cannot help but feel wistful and perhaps resentful.

People who survive cancer can seem like "winners," and people who are going to die of cancer, and those who have died, can seem like "losers." I hate that. It is not about being a winner or loser, it's about having good or bad luck. Luck is about randomness. Things happen randomly, and if these things are good, then that's good luck. If these things are bad, that's bad luck. People with good luck cannot take any credit for it. People with bad luck should not take it personally. Random events care nothing about what you deserve or don't deserve. Randomness does not reward some people and punish others.

Jenny was lucky. That's all there is to it. Gary and Jared were lucky. They did not have to lose her after all. Ideally, we would all be happy for them.

Try to take what you can from her story as you continue to live through your own. Perhaps some aspect of her story touched you or gave a new perspective on something you are dealing with. Certainly Jenny wanted the sharing of her story to have a positive impact on you. We hope it has.

Index